Madge

NOTHING TO MAKE A SHADOW

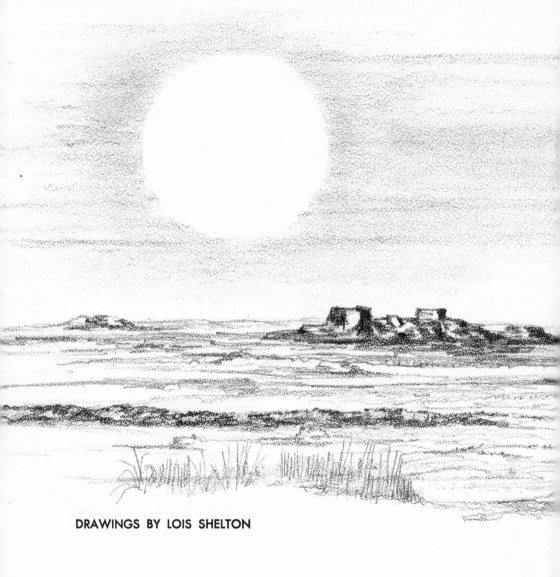

DRAWINGS BY LOIS SHELTON

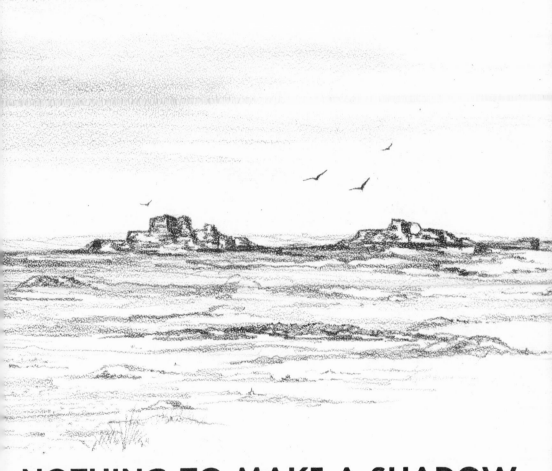

NOTHING TO MAKE A SHADOW

FAYE C. LEWIS

THE IOWA STATE UNIVERSITY PRESS / AMES / 1971

TO MALCOLM, ELIZABETH, AND VIRGINIA

FAYE CASHATT LEWIS, a native Iowan, was born in Carroll County, and migrated in childhood to the South Dakota she describes in this book. She was graduated from the University of South Dakota, Vermillion, and then obtained her degree in medicine from Washington University, St. Louis. Coming back to Iowa with her husband, also a physician, she lived in Kamrar from 1923–1928 and then moved to Webster City, where she has since made her home. After her children were grown, she was active in the practice of medicine from 1943–1969. Among the several books and articles about medical topics she has written are *Doc's Wife; Patients, Doctors and Families;* and *A Doctor Looks at Heart Trouble.* Her articles have appeared in *Atlantic, Today's Health, Alaska Sportsman,* and *Medical Economics,* and her verse and prose pieces in little magazines.

Library of Congress Cataloging in Publication Data

Lewis, Faye Cashatt.
    Nothing to make a shadow.

    1. Frontier and pioneer life—South Dakota.
I. Title.
F656.L4   917.83'03'3   73–171172
ISBN 0–8138–0775–1

Composed and printed by
The Iowa State University Press

First edition, 1971

First publication of Chapter Six in *Hinterland,* as "Rural Fourth,"
and of Chapter Twelve in *Prairie Schooner,* as "*Cimex Lectularius.*"

CONTENTS

Preface *vii*

1   The Leave-taking   *3*

2   Natives and Strangers   *11*

3   To the End of the Railroad   *17*

4   Wagon Trail to a New Home   *25*

5   Days of Serenity   *37*

6   Dakota Fourth   *48*

7   The Sod House Family   *57*

8   Our English Friends   *66*

9   Graces and Diversions   *70*

10 Pioneer Spirituality   *79*

11 Helping Uncle Grant Get a Farm   *86*

12 Torturings and Frustrations   *94*

13 First School   *100*

14 The Glory Tree   *107*

15 The Preacher Ladies   *119*

16 The Tumor Victims   *125*

17 Hazards and Shadows   *131*

18 The Bone Man   *138*

19 Chautauqua   *143*

20 Accessory Pioneers   *148*

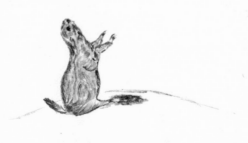

PREFACE

SOME PARTS of this book were written nearly forty years ago; none of it, however, during the time these recorded events were happening nearly seventy years ago. The only diary I kept was the one in my mind, never a written one. There is seldom much glamour in the everydayness of living, especially to the young. The young person, if he thinks abstractly of his mode of life at all, summarizes it as "the way things are," without further cogitation. It is the looking backward after a lapse of time that gives one perspective, enables one to assess the meanings and values of what he has lived through.

Thus it was only after I had grown up and moved away from South Dakota and began meeting people with a variety of backgrounds, most of them different from mine, that I came to realize I had had experiences shared by few of my contemporaries. My first writing about them was done for Quill Club, a writers' club in my home town, of which I have been a member for many years. Whenever it was my turn to read a paper, I could usually think of something to tell them about South Dakota. Two of these papers were published in little literary magazines.

The impetus to write a book about these homesteading days in South Dakota came when my children were still small. I could see that their lives were to be very different from either their father's or mine. It seemed the duty of both of us to give them a better understanding of themselves by enlightening them as best we could about the backgrounds from which they had come. The stories their paternal grandparents told gave them some knowledge of their heritage on their father's side—childhoods in England, Ireland and Wales; coal mines in Wales; steel mills in Pittsburgh, Pennsylvania, Indiana Harbor, Indiana, and Granite City, Illinois; the rigors of clearing farm land in Michigan's northern peninsula. These contrasting memoirs of the plains country must be my contribution. "With this mixed heritage, you could be anything," I wrote them encouragingly in one preface to the projected book.

I should not have believed that three books were to intervene between that time and this. Thus do contemporary pressures elbow aside more leisurely contemplations. When my latest book was in press I came to realize that this might go on and on, one thing after another replacing what I wanted to do most. So when my editor wrote me asking what next I had in mind I told him that this Dakota manuscript must take precedence over anything else.

A writer should never put off for too long writing a book that is especially meaningful to him. Things can happen to take most of the pleasure out of it, as have happened to me. There are now not many people left to share with me an intimate joy in it. My parents are dead, my two brothers and my sister, Marie. After the manuscript was in the mail, I suffered still another loss. I received word of Katherine's death. If the book had not been finished, I wondered for a time whether I should have had the heart to go on with it.

What I have said about Katherine as my close and long-time friend is limited by the time span of the book, and does not do her full justice. Her influence on this Dakota country burgeoned with the years. She, Katherine Ellis Kositzsky, was the first white person I knew to take an enlightened, humane attitude toward our Indians. To the settlers, these Sioux whose lands we were usurping, were savages, recent enemies. We scarcely thought of them as people, much less as a people with an indigenous culture of their own. Katherine lived for most of her married life in Winner, county seat of Tripp County. She made many friends among the Indians, for whose interests she worked tirelessly throughout her lifetime. She was a friend to them in the genuine sense of the word, not a condescending benefactor. She kept Indian young people in her home at times, to enable them to attend high school. Indian friends as well as white attended her funeral services, and one of the officiating pastors was the Reverend Broken Leg, a Sioux. Thinking remorsefully of all our ignorance, injustice, and cruelty toward the Indians, I like to believe that Katherine's benignity has conferred upon the rest of us some expiatory grace.

Thus there are many sadnesses connected with the publication of this book, but I have been able to persuade myself that I must not let them deter me. I lived for a time in one of the last new lands on this continent. Who is left to tell, if I do not, what it was like to live in a spot uncrowded and unpolluted, where solitudes transcended loneliness to become precious nurturings for the human spirit?

"There's nothing to make a shadow," mother said.
"If we could just see some shade somewhere,
it wouldn't seem quite so hot."

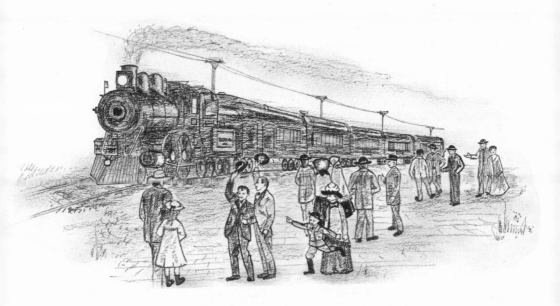

1 / THE LEAVE-TAKING

THIS LAST DAY OF SCHOOL was different from any other last day
that had ever been. It had been crowded to the background in
all our minds by the events looming in our immediate future,
thus having all the holiday enchantment squeezed out of it.

"What will our Dakota school be like?" I asked father at
the breakfast table.

"There isn't any school yet, where we are going," he replied.

Whereupon my two younger brothers burst into giggles of
delight and disbelief. Father was a quiet, serious man, not
much given to making a joke. But this must surely be one, they
were thinking.

I, who was thirteen, knew it was not a joke. I recognized
it as still another facet of the disruption taking place in our lives,
causing Mother to be both anticipatory and frightened, in turn.

I took two books back to the school library that morning,
Les Miserables and *The Shepherd of the Hills*. My feeling toward
books at that time was an indiscriminate hunger with no refinements of taste or appetite. I gorged on everything. My mind
was like a huge roll of recording tape, mostly blank, eager to be
impressed with any exposure. I had found these two volumes almost equally satisfying, edged slightly in favor of *Les Miserables*,
perhaps, because it was longer.

Our school library books were kept in a sectional bookcase
in one corner of the high school study hall. This was the first

year I had had access to them. There were still some I had not read, I thought regretfully, as I placed these two on their proper shelves. One fat volume, *The Newcomes,* I picked up and fingered once more. I had taken it home earlier in the year, but mother had made me return it, repeating sternly a former admonition that I should not bring such big books home. I read too late on too many nights when I had them.

I had learned to be careful not to say much to father about any books I was reading. He objected to novels, lumping them all as trash. I think he had never read one. "You should read books that are true, so they will teach you something," he would say to me. I knew, even then, how truth can strike like lightning from the pages of a novel, but I could not explain it to him.

We spent our last night at the home of the Roderick cousins, and Grandma Roderick got up early the next morning to fix us a lunch to eat on the train—fried chicken, bread and butter, young radishes, and onions from her garden. She was not our grandmother by blood. Mother's lovely sister, Edna, whom none of us children had known, had married Grandma Roderick's son, George, borne him two fine sons, then died three weeks after the birth of twins. Grief over this tragedy was never completely assuaged in our family, even by time, and for years the name Edna connoted beauty, love, and sadness to me.

We wore our good clothes on this train trip. In those days no trip was a casual affair; it was an occasion, calling for respectful recognition in clothing and deportment. The four-year-old twins had long-waisted dresses of dark red China silk. The boys had new suits, with knickers. Fern's were bloused evenly and neatly at the knees, but on Floyd's sturdy legs one buckle would not fasten, so the lower bands hung helter skelter on him at levels varying with his activity of the moment. I wore my first tailored suit, made by Mrs. Gibson, a local dressmaker. It was a rough brown wool, with pockets in the jacket, and a high-collared, striped, brown and gold silk waist.

After breakfast the boys went outside to play. Floyd was walking on the railing of the front porch and slipped off, pulling part of a clematis vine down with him, and tearing a three-cornered snag in the left knee of his knickers. He had started to cry, as a matter of policy, when he came in, but when he saw that father was in the back yard visiting with a neighbor and paying no attention to him, he was soon laughing and wriggling as mother pulled off his knickers to mend them. Floyd's clothes were always suffering damages. Once he wore a new navy blue cap with a white celluloid visor to Sunday school, and came home with little indentations bitten neatly into the celluloid, giving it the appearance of a nutmeg grater.

Our train was due at a quarter to ten. "There will be a big crowd down at the depot this morning," Grandma Roderick said. "All the neighbors around here plan to go, and most of our church people will be there. Everybody hates so much to see you leave."

She was talking to mother at the time, but mother modestly passed the complimentary implications along to father, genuinely unaware that any of them could be meant for her. "I know they will miss him in the church," she said, "and in a business way, too."

Father was superintendent of the Sunday school, and was depended upon in many ways as a lay worker in the church. He was fair and honest and not easily swayed, and his word carried a weight wherever it was spoken. He was in business with a senior partner, and the sign AYRHART AND CASHATT, GENERAL MERCHANDISE, was a proud and prominent one on Main Street. Father was usually the tallest in any crowd, with a thin, angular frame, and hair so thick it was always somewhat unruly. He was quiet almost to the point of taciturnity, and rather sad looking. I still see my father in the figure of my son, which, it seems to me, is all anyone should ask of immortality.

One person certain to be at the depot to see us off was Margaret Mozena. She wrote the Dedham news for the weekly *Coon Rapids Enterprise,* and met every passenger train that stopped. Notebook in hand, she inquired where all travelers were going and where they had come from. A number of stories were told about her, illustrating how assiduously she attended to her job. One Saturday night she was doing some shopping in Pfister's store when she heard the whistle of the ten o'clock flier. Immediately she detected a difference in the noise the train was making. It was slowing down for a stop! Some special passenger must be arriving. The train never picked up passengers in Dedham, and never stopped for anyone who had boarded this side of Chicago. Before the clerk could wrap up the length of hair ribbon she was buying for a niece, Margaret had snatched up her purse and was running down the street to the depot. The train had made its momentary stop before she arrived, but she was in time to see its one debarking passenger get into Doctor DeArmond's Reo, and while the doctor was cranking his car she had learned the visitor's name and that he was from Pittsburgh. Apparently he had been too startled to refuse this much information, but by the time she asked his business he had become cagier and made some vague reply about looking at some farmland. It was rumored later that he was interested in the local bank but did not want any publicity about it.

We walked to the depot, our luggage being brought by the

drayman and his team of mules. Many of our townspeople had already arrived. Margaret Mozena was there, getting a rich harvest of notes about Sunday visits at Coon Rapids and Viola Center, business trips to Omaha, expected summertime company in various households. The people clotted in changing groups about mother and father, while the twins and the boys romped about, indoors and out, with other children.

I avoided these adult groups, as they tended to become emotional, which was always painful to me. Being something of a recluse at that age, I wandered about in the background, watching the people. My classmates were all older and there was no feeling of intimacy between me and any of them.

I had already said my most important farewells and cared very little whether anyone here told me goodbye or not. I had walked past the schoolhouse at dusk on the evening before, and looked up at the windows of the rooms where Miss Bruce and Miss Willy taught. They were older than my parents, and getting gray-haired. Pretty soon they would die, and I should never see them again. There wasn't any school in Dakota, father had said. How would I learn to be a teacher? I remained numb and unmoved as these thoughts went through my mind.

I had slipped back into our house after they had taken the last of the furniture out. My feet made a hollow sound as I walked across the linoleum-covered floor to the north window of the dining room, and looked out at the diagonal path across old Mr. Strawl's weedy back yard. It was our shortcut to down town. "I must remember this," I told myself solemnly, "I'll never see it again." Thus was beginning my new awareness that there is a last time for everything; that familiar things may disappear and be gone forever. Mr. Strawl was a bachelor and he lived here with his fat old dog, a mongrel combination of several kinds of hound. The dog was never known to bark. A low growl was the only sound he ever made, apparently more communicative than menacing in intent. He was lying on the back step now, in the sun.

On my way over to the Roderick house I had stopped to sit for awhile on the long unused steps to the deserted Church of God. I often came here when I had something serious to think about. These steps, and the railing beside them, were overgrown with a tangle of wild morning glories. I loved them. They were so dense they made a shielding curtain of privacy to anyone who sat there. (It was years later that I first heard the hideous name "bindweed" applied to them, which I instantly rejected and tried to forget.)

On one occasion I had stopped here in the middle of March,

while it was still winter, when the vines left clinging to the railing were dismal brown wisps, blowing in the cold wind, and
the ones on the steps were covered deeply with snow. It was on
the day my twin sisters were born, and I was on my way home
from school at noon, half afraid to go on. I had told everybody
what a wonderful event had occurred at our house. Now I was
wondering whether I had not dreamed it, and might perhaps
have to go back this afternoon and face the ridicule of my classmates.

I had leaned against the railing with my back to the wind
and my mittens sheltering my face, trying to understand how
such a miracle could be true. They were the first twins I had
ever known in infancy; in fact, this was the first time the word
had ever been defined concretely for me. There were the
Roderick twins, but they were a boy and a girl, about my own
age, and I had never noticed anything different about them. But
these two little girl dolls, lying side by side in mother's bedroom
they were warm and breathing; I had touched them. They must
be real! Reassured, and fully convinced, I ran the rest of the
way home, getting my overshoes full of snow when I took a shortcut through the ditch at the edge of the street.

This train trip would be different than any I had taken before, since we were going west this time. My several previous
trips had all been eastward. Any train trip was an exciting and
enjoyable adventure. Once I had gone to the state fair in Des
Moines with father. We had to change trains at Madrid, where
we sat in the depot and ate crackers and cheese for lunch. It
was at the fair that I saw Negroes for the first time. "How do
they feel to be black when almost everyone else is white?" I had
asked father. "O, they must get used to it," father had replied,
vaguely.

Years later my understanding was supplemented greatly
when I attended medical school, the only girl in a class of fifty.
I was able to do my work in the laboratories and listen to the
lectures without undue strain, even with enjoyment. It was
when I was called upon to recite in class that I felt painfully
pinpointed. I used to think, "My girl voice is like a black skin
in a roomful of whites."

My other train trips had been for summer vacations at Little
Grandma's house in Coon Rapids, the next town east. I had
made the most recent two of these trips alone, which gave me a
satisfying feeling of importance never lessened throughout my
stay. I adored Little Grandma, and her tiny brown house with
the weeping willow tree in front, and her garden bordered by
cherry trees was a shrine to me. She could think of endless ways

to delight me, such as letting me set the table for the two of us, cook on her kitchen range in a toy skillet, catch fireflies—lightning bugs to us—with the neighbor children. The cherries were just beginning to ripen one summer when I arrived, and she had tied a rhubarb leaf over the first cherry on a new little tree, to save it for me from the robins. On one of my earliest visits she told me I might pick some peonies—she called them pinies—to put in a vase in the house. I came back in a few moments, both hands full of gorgeous peony heads, which I tumbled proudly onto the kitchen table.

An aunt who was present, whose name I have forgotten—probably a Freudian rejection—exclaimed, "But you've ruined them! You haven't left them any stems!"

Little Grandma looked at me and said quickly, "But these will be very pretty in a special kind of vase. I know just what we can put them in."

She stood on a kitchen chair and brought down from the top shelf of the cupboard a squat old gravy boat of ironstone china with gold leaves on it. Even the dwarfed stems of my peonies could reach the water level in this vessel, and their tousled heads of red, pink, and white filled the boat and drooped over its sides, making a pretty if unusual arrangement. Little Grandma set the bouquet on the center table in the parlor, beside the green plush-covered album and the framed daguerreotype of my grandfather whom I had never seen, in his Civil War uniform. From that moment on, I knew I should love Little Grandma forever. The word "grandma" became a very special one in my lexicon, ranking with "Christmas," "ice cream," and "Jesus."

I had been wandering about the waiting room watching the people and listening to snatches of conversation. Mother was sitting in a corner with three other women, and from the worried little frown on her face I knew they were talking again about the dangers that threatened us in this new country. "Just don't listen to such talk," father had told her more than once in these past few weeks, but her vulnerability must have been apparent in her face, for she seemed unable to escape this scaremongering.

Prairie fires and rattlesnakes were favorite topics in these conversations, but now they were talking about Indians, I noted as I sat down near them. "You know the Indians up there are the Sioux," one woman, a teacher, was saying, "and all the history books say they are very warlike."

Concern for these distant dangers was now replaced by attention to hazards nearer at hand. As train time drew nearer the children were becoming more and more excited and restless.

They were running out to look at the signal tower, gaze down the track, lay their ears against the rails to catch the first reverberations, walking on the rails, running in again to look at the clock on the waiting room wall. The air was filled with parental admonitions. "Don't go out on the tracks any more. You know a train can come awfully fast—fifty miles an hour, sometimes." "Don't stand too close when it comes in, or you could be sucked under the wheels." "Remember poor Dutch who had his leg cut off by a train."

The first distant whistle of the steam locomotive was an electrifying sound that no one could have disregarded. We were all on our feet in an instant, surging through the door. Facing the approaching monster, eyes fixed, mouths agape, almost breathless, we felt the tremors under our feet ascend throughout our whole bodies. Then, when the train came to a panting standstill, there were the quick movings aside and forward that separated our family of seven, somehow, from the rest of the crowd and lifted us to the platform of the car, where mother and father and I turned for one last look and final gestures of farewell to the waving crowd below. The boys had run ahead of us into the coach, and the twins clung to my hands, too frightened by all the excitement to know where to look.

The twins and I had one of the red plush-covered seats, with mother and father behind us and the boys across the aisle. The bell clanged, and the train moved forward. The window beside us was open, a layer of dust and fine cinders on the sill. I leaned out to take a backward look, not at anyone or anything in particular, just at the place we were leaving. "Don't get yourself dirty on that window," mother admonished, too late. When I sat back in my seat there were smudges on both hands and wrists. The conductor, a kindly elderly man in blue uniform and gold-braided cap, came to take our tickets from father, and patted both twins on the head causing them to shrink against me in shy confusion.

The train was now going faster. There was something inexorable in the steady, powerful clank of the wheels. I felt caught up in a power from which there was no escape. I sank against the seat, my body relaxed but my mind still in a turmoil. I rubbed my hands together trying to get the grime off them lest my new suit be soiled. I had worn it only twice before, both times to Sunday school.

I looked down at my suit now, seeing in it a new importance. It seemed an integral part of what was happening to me. Looking at this, my first young-lady outfit, I could not imagine ever again going barefoot down to the Brushy to fish and wade and sail little boats. Nor to Minnich's pasture in the fall after school to gather hazel nuts, which I had been able to carry home by the flour-sackful as so much of the bulk of them was light-weight husks. Nor could I see myself, ever again, climbing the Duchess apple tree in our back yard to shake down the fruit which the boys and I and the neighbors' children started eating in its green state from the time the apples were not much larger than marbles. My hair was changed, too, to go with the suit. I noticed it every time I turned my head. My long braids were no longer flying free behind me or caught up with ribbons in the back. They were now wound around my head and pinned, making it feel heavy and aching.

An unknown blankness, dotted with hazards, was all I could see before us. No school in Dakota. Not even any books except the few we were taking with us, and I had read all of them except the Bible, more than once. Maybe no one but Indians for neighbors, and they would not like us. When would I see Little Grandma again? Little Grandma was old, I realized suddenly. I had never thought of it before. But she must be; she was my father's mother. She must be older, even, than Miss Bruce and Miss Willy, and would probably die sooner than they did. My emotions succumbed to this final bombardment. I felt a choking in my throat, and my eyes began to sting.

As I took the handkerchief from the pocket of my jacket, mother leaned forward to ask solicitously, "Are you getting that dust in your eyes?"

I nodded without turning to look at her, easing my conscience with the thought that I had only gestured, not spoken, the lie.

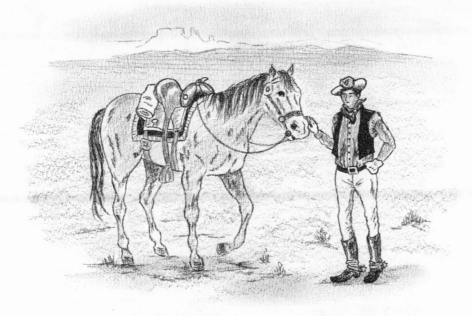

2 / NATIVES AND STRANGERS

NOT MANY PEOPLE know there is a Dallas in South Dakota. Cross country travelers may take brief note of it as a small dot on the road map, a possible source of emergency food and gasoline, or shelter for the night if the hour is late. It is a quiet town now, somnolent and resigned, its dreams of grandeur withered long ago. But it was once vibrant with these dreams, rocked with explosive ambitions. In its livelier days there was probably more exuberance per capita in Dallas than in any other place in the country. The Gateway to the Rosebud, it was called, the gathering and dispersal point for people who came to take advantage of the opening of the Rosebud Indian Reservation to white settlement. This was almost the last frontier country of our West, a last chance to get a homestead in government land hitherto unoccupied.

Our Midwest offers few endpoints of interest for tourists. Most of them consider it a wide monotonous area to be traveled through, at all permissible speed, to the more scenic areas on either side. Three of these itinerants were in the little Dakota restaurant where my husband and I stopped for lunch several summers ago; a man and a woman probably in their mid-thirties, and a boy about ten years old. They were well along in their meal when we entered and were seated at a table beside them. The man was eating steadily; not with any apparent enthusiasm, but as a methodical person getting on with the next order of business. The boy, too, was attacking his hamburger without

11

dalliance, and chewing with apparent gusto. The woman, how-ever, had a restless, critical little frown on her face as she looked at the food on her plate, a thick slice of meat loaf and a hump of mashed potatoes with pale gravy running down the sides. She had eaten very little of it.

"What on earth do people in this country eat for vitamins?" she asked in an exasperated undertone.

"What other excuse is there for this stuff?" her husband replied, paddling his fork in his small side dish of stewed toma-toes islanded with pulpy masses of bread.

The woman shuddered. "Honestly, how people out here live——."

Her husband pushed back his plate and lit a cigarette.

"You're so darned critical, Carol, of things you don't know anything about," he said in a weary voice. "One reason they don't have more here is the grasshoppers. This spot was just about the grasshopper metropolis of the world a few years ago. They ate everything but the people and the cattle."

"Then why do they go on living here? Why don't they leave?"

"Maybe they like their own houses," offered the boy.

"It's lucky for us that a few of them stayed," the man said, "or we shouldn't be having anything to eat this noon at all."

"Then perhaps we'd have flown over this spot, as I wanted to," the woman said, "instead of crawling over it like this."

"We were doing eighty for awhile this morning; I saw the speedometer," defended the boy.

"Give me one of those," the woman said, indicating her husband's cigarette.

"But you haven't eaten anything," he protested.

"All I'm going to."

She took the proffered cigarette and went over to the counter where a miscellaney of oddments were displayed.

"Have you any postcards?" she asked of the young man who came in from the kitchen to attend her.

He took a cardboard box from the glass showcase.

"No, not picture postcards," she said, impatiently. "Just plain postcards."

"You'll have to get those at the post office," he told her.

"Wait! What are those pictures of?"

He offered her the box again. "Just local views, and scenery."

She picked up one of the cards. "Views? Of what?"

"Of the town," he said, flushing, "and the Three Buttes you'll come to, a little farther west, and just the prairie."

Something about the young man seemed to have roused her

interest. She picked up two of the cards at random, laid a coin on the counter, and then lingered a moment as he arranged the others in piles again and returned them to the box.

"Have you lived here long?" she asked him.

"I don't live here except in the summer. I teach school in the East the rest of the year."

"You mean you come here for vacations?" Her voice was shrill with astonishment.

The young man shielded his embarrassment with a defensive dignity.

"I like it here," he said quietly. "I'm afraid I couldn't explain why."

He excused himself with a courteous little half-bow, and returned to the back room. She stood staring after him for a few moments, and then walked slowly back to her table, where her husband and son were eating lemon pie. She waved aside her husband's offer to order some dessert for her, her eyes fixed, apparently without visual impression, on the picture of a Sioux Indian on a calendar on the wall, her restless, mobile face retaining its expression of puzzled wonderment.

"Reginald," she said, as her husband arose and picked up the check, "who do you suppose he is?"

"Who?"

"The young man I was talking to."

"How should I know? Unless he's the writer the proprietor told me was staying here. Some kind of poet, I believe he said."

The woman's face cleared. A poet! That seemed to explain everything to her. The three of them left, and we never saw them again.

The young man remained in my mind, too. I asked our waitress about him, but she said she was new there, and could tell me only that he was visiting the owner, maybe a relative, and that he came back every summer. She didn't know his name, only that they called him Jim. I sent her to ask if I might talk to him, but he had left the restaurant and gone to the ranch house, several miles away. I never saw him again, either. He must have had some early connection with this country, I mused, to bring him back year after year. His name might even be familiar to me, as one of the roots in my own past. However it had come about, I felt certain that he was one of us who look at Dakota with eyes of love.

I feel a great pity for anyone who does not have a romantic era tucked away somewhere in his past; a time on neutral ground between myth and reality to which the mind may turn for refreshment and inspiration. Such a time is a stabilizer between a too idealistic youth and the harshnesses of mature understanding. As one grows older such periods of enjoyment take on greater values, until in time they make a precious rosary for the mind, which counts each bead against a score of disappointments and bitternesses, telling itself with a hectic fierceness, "Whatever else may come, however soon all may end, these delights, at least, I have had."

Just such a romantic era was our homesteading experience, hardships and all. And the peculiar thing about it is the fact that we recognized it as such at the time. The lives of so many of us are made up of a youth spent in looking forward to utopias that never come, and an old age given to reflections upon past joys that we did not recognize when we had them, that it is refreshing to remember that for one brief period we took life as it came, and found it good.

When I say "we" I mean my brothers and sisters and I. If our parents had kept diaries and set down faithfully each day's happenings, the result would probably have been a truer account than this one of mine. Yet, what is truth? Is it only events? Are not feelings a part of it? As they recorded the day's labors, the deprivations, the droughts and disappointments, all the harshnesses of their lives, could they have balanced the equation sufficiently with the hopes and dreams and satisfactions to make it equal happiness, in the telling? If not, then it would not have been the truth, for we were happy.

In their early childhood three of my grandsons with their parents lived for a time in a state of great deprivation, bordering on actual want. Not many of the details were divulged to their grandparents at the time. We were shielded from the truth. It was only later, when their circumstances had changed to comfort, even opulence, that occasional facts trickled through to us. They were painful enough to us, even in the past tense. Our own grandchildren going hungry, wearing rags! This was something we could not bear to think about, much less talk about.

Then one day last winter my husband and I had lunch with these grandsons, all now in their teens. Their conversation turned upon that year they had lived on the beach. The three of them— Jeff, Sid, and Tim—chattered away with great gusto, all through the lunch hour, telling anecdotes and memories of that year. And the central theme running through all this talk was how much fun they had had! Swimming, fishing, catching shrimp, playing games on the beach, digging caves in the sand dunes—not a word of remembered hardship, no bitterness over their deprived state. My husband and I listened to them with amazement and great relief. We were convinced that whatever stringencies they had suffered had been superficial and temporary, leaving no scars. Here was one retroactive worry that could be erased from our minds forever.

Similarly, these homesteading days in South Dakota that are so pleasurable to me in the recalling would look much different to many other people, perhaps to most other people. In connection with the present much touted war on poverty, I have thought that we might have been considered eligible for some federal beneficence if it had existed at that time, and if anyone had known about us. I have wondered many times what my father's reaction would have been if a government agent had knocked at the door of our claim shack and asked him if he would like to be enrolled in some federal relief program. Father always kept his shotgun standing behind the kitchen door. On such an occasion I think he might have made a few gestures with it. Low as an appraisal of our material status might have rated us, we still considered ourselves among the haves of the world. Our riches were good health, ambition, hope, and pride. So much pride! I think my father was the proudest man I knew, and his pride infected and bolstered us all. We considered ourselves people of importance.

One who seeks a true account of the early days in this prairie country could not do better than to go to the college campus at Brookings, South Dakota, and look at the paintings of Harvey Dunn on permanent display there. Here is the whole story—canvases depicting the vastness, the loneliness, the desolation—and surmounting it all, the serenity and joy in "The Prairie is My Garden." This last picture shows the spirit of the prairie frontier, the how and why of all the endurance.

My copy of "The Prairie is My Garden" was a gift from my sister-in-law, Hazel. I had never seen the picture before. It came in a cardboard mailing tube and lay on the counter in our office drug room for several days before any attention was paid to it, among a pile of drug samples and advertising matter, which was what I thought it was—an ad from a drug firm. (Not that all drug ads are regarded as trash. It could have been one of the much prized Geigy calendars, for instance, with twelve breath-taking views of Swiss scenery.) When I finally noticed the return address I knew it was a personal item, and took it home with me.

When I drew it out of the mailing tube and unrolled it, I groped for a chair and sat down. My hands were trembling, and I had a mildly hallucinatory feeling. Or was it *déjà vu?* Was not this my mother in her young years, standing in the foreground? No, it looked more like my niece, Velma. But the buildings were surely those on our homestead. No, the positions of the house and barn were transposed, as in the negative of a snapshot. The creek was too near the house. There were no buttes visible in the west. It was only after shuffling all these facts about in my mind that I was convinced this was not 'our old home on the claim, somehow magically resurrected, but someone else's home, beloved as ours was. For the painting radiated the magic of love and enchantment that flows from the mind and suffuses the material environment in its glow.

I told a friend about my new picture and that I wanted to get it framed for its own protection, as I had already unrolled it so many times to look at it that the edges were getting frayed.

"Take it to the Irvine Paint Shop in Ames," she told me. "There's a woman in there who will know exactly what to do with it."

I did so, and Mrs. Irvine, in turn, unrolled it and looked at it. "Ah!" she said softly, " 'The Prairie is My Garden.' I have that picture hanging in my house where I can see it as soon as I get up in the morning."

Another one of us! Another child of the prairie country, to whom the prairie would always mean home, in its most soulful sense. We exchanged data about our respective pasts. Her father had been a minister in northern Nebraska, less than a hundred miles from where we had lived.

3 / TO THE END OF THE RAILROAD

An old vaudeville joke had a comedian say, "I want to go to Chicago the worst way." And his partner replied, "Then take the Milwaukee."

It was the Milwaukee we took that long-ago day in 1909 from Dedham, Iowa, to go to Dallas, making a change at Omaha to the Northwestern. To my brothers and me, one of the special thrills of this train trip was that we would be going almost to the end of the line. The railroad extended only two stations west of Dallas. We had no premonition of it then, but the "end of the line" was in sight for most railroads, in a symbolic sense. I am one who regrets this very much. My young grandson expressed amazement when I wanted to stop to look at an old steam railroad engine being preserved in a town park.

"It's a very romantic sight to me," I told him.

"What could be romantic about an old steam engine?" he asked, incredulously.

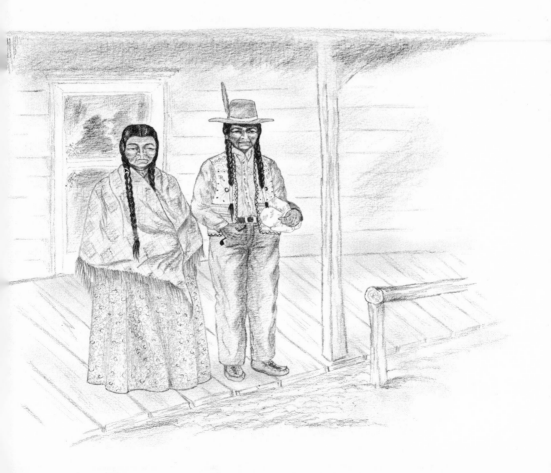

"Do you remember the first time you came to visit us by yourself," I tried to explain, "and you had to change planes at O'Hare? You said it was thrilling to you to see people taking off for Rome, Cairo, Bangkok. That's the same kind of feeling I used to have waiting for a train."

My regret over the demise of our passenger trains is not merely a sentimental, nostalgic feeling, however. It is a practical assessment of values. In my opinion no kind of travel over land areas offers more possibilities of luxury than does the train. In luxury, its only competitor is the steamship. It seems to me foolish and unnecessary for trains to try to compete with airplanes on the basis of speed; they will never make a good showing on that comparative basis. But with some studied effort they should be able to attract a livelihood-sustaining business from present travel in private cars. The beautiful convenience of travel in one's own car is being eroded away as a consequence of its own excellence. Parking is becoming a more and more frustrating dilemma; city traffic becomes increasingly congested and hazardous; our network of freeways grows in complexity, offering maximum in speed, minimum in pleasure. Closeness to the country is being lost; interesting little villages have become endpoints of exits, never seen. All this makes cross-country touring by car no longer the pleasure it once was.

I have been gratified, occasionally, to read of others who think as I do that we are depriving ourselves of many benefits by allowing our railroads to pass into desuetude. The sum of these opinions has finally been sufficiently weighty to make its influence felt and to result in some action. The early AMTRAK trains are now rolling, and I hope they continue to roll along increasingly diversified routes.

These ideas are not the fabric of a daydream. They are demonstrable facts in some other places. One summer I accompanied my husband on a hunting trip to British Columbia. While he was out in the wilds, I set out to see some of the country. I went from Kamloops to Vancouver by bus, and by steamship to Victoria. On my return trip, I went by train back to Kamloops. Omitting Victoria, the endpoint of my visit and one of the most charming cities on our continent, no day's travel I have ever had surpassed my journey on the Canadian Pacific from Vancouver to Kamloops. The car I rode in had windows cut low, almost to the floor, giving the maximum view. Our seats were upholstered armchairs easily moved about to one's convenience. There we lounged about throughout the daylight hours of an entire day, free of the fatigue of driving and watching traffic, no decisions to make about stops or routes, food and ·

drink at hand, with room to stir about and change positions, and our route along the beautiful Fraser valley traversed some of the most magnificent mountain scenery in the world, in the Canadian Rockies. An added boon was my conversation with some Canadian citizens. For much of this ride, a businessman from Kamloops was seated in a chair on my left, and on my right was a woman who lived in a town just west of Kamloops. They knew the route well, and throughout the day a live brew of conversation took place among the three of us, mostly questions from me and information about the country from my pleasant and entertaining companions. All this contributed to what I call luxury in traveling.

However, little of a luxurious nature happened on our trip to Dallas that long-ago day—only the excitement inherent in the fact of our going. But luxury was not a part of our lives anyway, so we did not miss it. We enjoyed watching other passengers, looking at the scenery, the glimpses we had of all the little towns where we stopped. The boys made frequent excursions up and down the aisles investigating everything—the toilets, the water cooler, the tipping of the seat backs up and down, the working of the windows. Mother remarked that some of the windows in that coach would work better than they had in many a day, after the limbering up the boys gave them. At noon there was a hearty meal from the market basket full of food supplied us by Grandma Roderick; a new kind of picnic, enjoyable if somewhat messy, accompanied by much licking of fingers.

The sun had set by the time we reached Dallas, and the coolness of the evening had begun. We were to learn that this was a characteristic of this country. However hot it was during the day, the nights almost invariably were cool.

Many people were milling about the depot platform as we stepped off the train, many more than had come to see us off at Dedham. Somehow we were not surprised. Were we not coming to one of the most important places in the country? "Little Chicago" Dallas had already been nicknamed by some of its boosters.

Passengers had been dribbling off the train at each stop after leaving Norfolk, Nebraska. Now most of the remaining ones disembarked with us. It looked as though not more than a half-dozen were left, to go on to Colome and Winner. The people waiting on the platform had come to meet friends and relatives, to inquire about shipments of household goods, or to join in the excitement of welcoming the new people. No one could have felt lonely or unwanted in that crowd. Everyone was being greeted. "Stranger" was a warm and inclusive word, almost synonymous with "friend."

"Where are you from, stranger?" "Got a place to stay tonight?" "Need any help loading your goods in the morning?" "Glad to see you, and the missus will want to meet you, too."

Not knowing anybody in this new country had been a serious drawback to mother's enthusiasm for the move. While she never doubted father's veracity, it had been difficult for her to accept at face value his reassurances about how soon she would get acquainted. Now I could see a relieved belief easing the expression on her face, which communicated itself to me. Seeing mother worried was always painful to me, and I could usually detect the signs of it.

Mother and I and the twins stood beside the depot while father and the boys collected some luggage that had been checked. While we were waiting, the twins began raising quite a furor—squealing, crying out, dancing about. They were timid little creatures, afraid of a great many things, including insects. Now, as we stood under a light, we were beset by a host of large brown beetles. The boys, when they rejoined us, teased and made fun of the twins, but father tried to reassure them.

"They're only June bugs," he told them. "They don't bite, and they can't hurt you in any way."

Whereupon the twins quieted down, partly from reassurance but mostly from father's authoritative presence. None of us misbehaved when father was around. At the end of the month when mother tore a page off the calendar, remarking, "Well, this is the end of June; tomorrow is the first of July," Marjory squealed again, this time with delight, and said, "O, goody! Now the June bugs will have to go."

Carrying our suitcases, we started walking up the main street.

"Where are the Indians?" Fern asked.

"Look ahead of you," father replied with a chuckle.

Fern looked, and stopped still in his tracks until father nudged him on. Approaching, a few feet ahead of us, were an Indian man and a squaw. Both wore moccasins. Both wore their hair in braids. The squaw had a dark plaid blanket wrapped about her dumpy figure. The man wore a sleeveless beaded jacket over a dark shirt. Their faces were wrinkled, leathery, imperturbable. Fern was still dragging his feet as we met them, and the twins hid their faces against mother and me and stumbled as we pulled them along, half supporting them. Floyd, with his usual bravado, strode on ahead of the rest of us, and I thought there was a momentary flicker of something more than passivity on the squaw's face as we passed them.

Many of the "sidewalks" in Dallas were sandy paths. As we walked farther uptown we came to some boardwalks, still new and clean, as foot traffic over them left only traces of sand, not the sticky black mud we were accustomed to see in Iowa.

We were all hungry, and our first stop was to be at a restaurant. They had a fine one here, father said. "Fine" to him meant plenty of good plain food cooked according to his liking, not necessarily as a gourmet would prepare it. We had crossed the street to get to the restaurant and passed a harness shop on the way. From the open doorway a cowboy came out carrying a saddle, which he put on a bay pony tied to a hitching post in front.

"Had to get a belly strap sewed back on," he said to father. "Got it ripped plumb off at a ruckus out in Mellette County."

"Do you know him?" Floyd asked in a half-whisper, awe-struck.

"No," father said, "but that doesn't mean anything out here."

The cowboy was a glamorous figure to the boys and me, and, I suspected, somewhat so to mother and father. Hungry as we were, we lingered awhile in the restaurant doorway while he fastened the repaired saddle on his pony. A description of him would not sound glamorous. He was short and bowlegged, and there was nothing particularly attractive about his features. But he had a bright red kerchief knotted at his neck, his broad-rimmed felt hat was tilted just a little, there was a devil-may-care look on his face and a swagger to his walk, and his spurs jangled at every step. We watched until he mounted his pony and started down the street at a lope, acutely aware of the admiring stares following him.

And now, finally, to supper at the restaurant, where hungry customers were fed at two long, oilcloth-covered tables. One of them was now empty and being cleared of the used dishes, but a half-dozen people were still eating at the other table—all men. We drew out chairs and sat down. There were friendly "howdies" and other greetings from our tablemates, and they began passing dishes of food to us. But the waitress bringing our plates interposed, saying fresh food would be brought to us in a jiffy. The boys were looking slightly disgruntled, and mother asked them what was the matter.

"I never saw a restaurant like this," Floyd said.

"How many restaurants have you ever seen?" father asked, jokingly. "Five or six?"

We all knew what the trouble was, and I shared their disappointment, but would not say so. The kind of restaurant meal we had been expecting, and hoping for, was one served at little tables, with each person's food in little side dishes about his plate. Inexperienced as we were, we knew how things ought to be done in a restaurant. This was just like eating at home, except for the oilcloth; we always had a tablecloth; usually white. These features, objectionable to us, were the ones that had attracted father to the place. "Family style meals" was their advertising slogan. Father had his quirks about selecting eating places. I recalled how he would pick a place to eat when we went to the fair in Des Moines. He would walk through the dining area at the fair grounds looking at the screened, open-air dining rooms and pick one where he could see bowls of sliced ripe tomatoes on the tables.

We were served promptly with a generous platter of roast beef, and mashed potatoes, gravy, stewed tomatoes.

"There's corn, too," the waitress told us. "We ran out and had to open another can. It will be ready in a minute."

We all ate heartily except the twins. They picked at the food suspiciously, saying it didn't taste right, not like we had at home. They looked wistfully at the plate of cookies the waitress brought for dessert in lieu of the lemon pie which she said was all gone. But mother told them firmly that they couldn't have cookies until they had eaten their other food. Mother's firmness was always more effective when backed by father's presence, so the twins ate some more from their plates.

"This critter was never fed any corn," father said, taking another helping of beef. His remark was not critical in tone, only a statement of fact. Grass-fed beef was what one would expect in a prairie country. He was probably thinking it would be different when he and all the other new settlers had turned the grasslands into luxuriant cornfields. This was a part of the dreams.

"What do the Indians eat?" Fern asked.

Fern was a slow thinker; slow and thorough. He chewed all the nuances of meaning out of an idea before discarding it. It was evident that the Indians had remained in the back of his mind since meeting the two on the street, and he would keep on probing for further knowledge about them.

"The ones I've seen eating were eating the same food we were," father said. "I don't know what they eat at home, but I've heard they make stew out of dog meat."

"Did you eat with any Indians when you were up here before?" Fern asked, in astonishment.

"Once," father replied.

"In this restaurant?"

"No. It was in a little lunchroom down by the depot. Three Indians were sitting at the counter with me and one other white man."

Fern pondered this information thoughtfully. It would suggest further questions to be asked about father's two previous trips to this country; the first time to look at the land and make a selection from what was still available, and the second time, earlier this spring, to build the house and barn that were now ready for us.

It was dark outside by the time we had finished eating. The twins were yawning and rubbing their eyes.

"We ought to get these girls to bed pretty soon," mother said to father. "They haven't had anything but little catnaps all day."

"O, I'm not tired," Marjory protested. "I just look tired."

There was one hotel in town, one block farther up the street. Since being built a year ago it had already had one addition built onto it. The rooms were not yet numbered.

"We're giving you the big room in the middle, on the north side of the hall," the hotel clerk told father.

The room contained three double beds, an oak dresser, three straight chairs. The floor was of wide pine boards, with no covering and no finish on the wood. The partitions that separated our room from the room on each side were also of wide, unfinished pine boards, and they extended only part way to the ceiling, just high enough so that even a tall man like father could not see over them.

One unshaded electric light bulb lit the room. Accustomed as we were to kerosene lamps, this convenience, hung by a wire from the middle of the ceiling, was a very modern bit of luxury to us. Mother's fancy china parlor lamp, with red roses painted on it, was one of the things she had regretted leaving behind. But father had decreed it should be sold, along with many other possessions that were not strictly practical. Electric lighting for homes did not become common in this country until many years later. When I attended the university at Vermillion, the rooms in our dormitory were lighted by a refinement of this same drop cord from the ceiling method; the cords were much longer, and could be draped above a dresser anywhere in the room.

We all went to bed without delay, and father and mother were soon asleep. The twins, however, were restless and fretful. The boys began teasing them, which made them increasingly irritable. The occupants of the rooms on either side of us had now come in, and we could hear them talking and moving about.

"Listen!" Floyd hissed at the twins. "Do you know who's in those other rooms? They're Indians, and they'll jump over the walls and get you if you don't keep still!"

There was not another word out of the twins. They cowered to sleep beside me, and none of us woke until daylight.

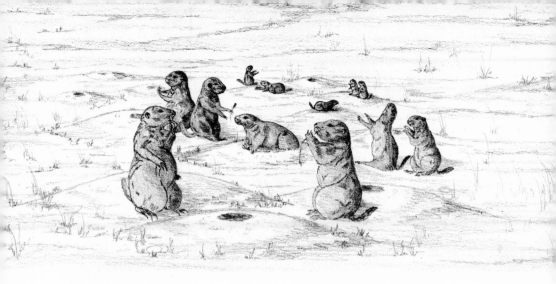

4 / WAGON TRAIL TO A NEW HOME

WE WERE UP AT DAYLIGHT. Father's idea of the purpose of daylight was to enable a man to see to do his work. Sleeping was for darkness only. "You must have got up early this morning," a neighbor once said to father, commenting on what he had accomplished in a half day.

"No," father said, apologetically, "it was nearly five o'clock."

We are told that children in their mature years often rebel against things that harassed them in childhood. As I grew away from parental discipline, one of the things I enjoyed was sleeping late whenever I could manage it. But I have never been able to exorcise completely the feeling of guilt that goes with it. This principle of father's about early rising was more than an adherence to the accepted code of living for the farmer of that day. With him it was an obsession, a fancied morality. He was an early-rise farmer, earlier than anyone else. To the rest of us it seemed a useless extreme, but we accepted it as we accepted all of father's dictates, without bothering to wonder what his "or else" would have been. Resentments did boil up in the boys and me on those occasions when we had to sit around for a while after breakfast, waiting until it was light enough to see to do the chores; but they boiled over into words only among ourselves, never in father's presence.

None of us wanted to sleep late on this morning, however. We were too full of eagerness and excitement. Father and the boys hurried to the depot after breakfast to see about the loading

25

of our household goods, leaving mother, the twins, and me to wander about, exploring the town. Dallas was three years old then, and growing rapidly. All the buildings were new, of course, many still unpainted, and many still in the process of being built. There were boardwalks to accommodate three blocks of the business district, the streets in the other parts of town being marked by paths and wagon tracks, with the grass not entirely worn off them.

We walked up and down the one main street, looking in shop windows, watching the people, many of whom greeted us warmly, like old friends. Everybody seemed exuberant and buoyed up by the prospects ahead of us, a new home on land of our own. Many of these people were property owners for the first time. Instant acquaintanceships were springing up all around us.

"What's your name?" "Where are you from?" "Where's your claim?" "Come to see us when we get our house built."

These exchanges took place whenever people stopped to talk, and that was as often as a look of friendliness was beamed in anyone's direction.

The only placid people on the streets were the Indians, dotted thickly among the crowds, interested spectators of the panorama and providing one of the most colorful aspects of it. They were the Sioux. It was said, however, that they preferred to be called the Dakotahs, as Dakotah meant friend, but I have always suspected that this was a euphemism of the history books.

The older men wore their hair in braids, like the squaws, but the young bucks had white-man haircuts. The squaws were all fat. They wore calico dresses, with large plaid wool shawls wrapped about them, hot as it was. Men, women, and children wore moccasins, and some of the men and boys had sleeveless beaded jackets like the one we had seen the evening before.

Having walked the length of the main street and back again, we learned that the largest general store in town was the one just across from our hotel. We went in it to look around. There was a display rack standing on a counter near the front of the store, with an assortment of hair switches hanging from it. An old Indian man was standing beside it, fingering the hair thoughtfully and caressingly. We watched him for awhile, but he paid no attention to us, and after we had strolled along toward the back of the store, mother said to me, half amused and half fearful, that she wondered if he was thinking of the good old scalping days now gone forever, she hoped. Being scalped by Indians was one of the three tragedies we had been most warned about by friends and relatives back home. The other two were being bitten by rattlesnakes and being burned up in a prairie fire.

Father and the boys joined us about midmorning, and there was a conference about the groceries we would need.

"Let's get some beefsteak, for one thing," Floyd suggested.

Father and mother both laughed. "Any fresh meat wouldn't be fit for the dog, if we had a dog, after we had carried it all the distance ahead of us in this heat," father said. "Bacon and ham will have to do for us until winter."

The same restrictions applied to our entire grocery list. No butter, cream, or fresh milk. Only staples that would not spoil in the heat could be considered. These included sugar, tea, coffee, flour, canned milk, canned corn and tomatoes, gallon pails of sorghum and corn syrup, potatoes, rice, eggs, and a few lemons for pie.

Our possessions had been loaded into two lumber wagons, one of them drawn by Pete Putnam's team of mules, and the other by our own Duke and Barney—white Duke and bay Barney —a heavy work team father had bought when he had come to build the house and barn. Pete was a neighboring homesteader whose claim was about a mile from ours. He had the teams and wagons waiting for us, and had borrowed an extra seat for our lumber wagon, for mother, the twins, and me. Father and the boys had the seat in front. The back of the wagon was piled full of our belongings, and Pete's wagon was also so full there was scarcely room for him to sit.

Now we began to have the real feeling of pioneers, setting out into a new country alone.

"O, I want to get where nobody in the whole world has ever been before!" Floyd said, ecstatically. I shared this feeling, but mother did not, and it was painful to her to hear us talk in this manner.

Our route took us south and west from Dallas, eighteen and a half miles. The first two thirds of the way was through Gregory County, "old" country, comparatively speaking. People had been living here for several years. At the south edge of Dallas we passed a little cemetery, a plot with a fence around it and still covered with virgin prairie grass. No trees, no flowers, not even any shrubs; just the dozen or so lonely looking headstones. Mother shuddered, and turned to look back at it as we passed.

"What a God-forsaken looking place!" she said. "I don't ever want to be buried there."

"Who thinks of burying?" father said. "People in this country don't die easy."

There were sprouting farmsteads along the way, becoming

sparser as we progressed. Tiny houses, barns and other outbuild-
ings, haystacks, fences, gardens, plowed fields showing some
green from spring plantings—homemakings of fiercely indomit-
able spirits. Many looked naked in their utter treelessness, others
had wisps of new groves on the north of the buildings, hopeful
dreams of future windbreaks against winter storms. These groves
—pines for hardiness, or cottonwoods for quick growth—illustrated better than anything else how tenuous were the chances
for survival of general farming in a country whose soil and rain-
fall were better adapted for grasses. They were frail; puny as
premature infants, which in cruelty had been uprooted from the
nursery. Some of the trees were already dead; none looked
vigorous. Could the hopeful determination of the settlers pre-
vail against all the adverse odds? Time would tell.

We plodded along, no faster than a man could walk. Duke
and Barney were built for the heavy work of the plow, not for
speed. Pulling a lumber wagon, even an empty one, is not a
lightweight job, and our two wagons were loaded. The horses
never once broke into a trot, and father would not have permitted them to continue it if they had. Plop, plop, was the noise
their broad hoofs made on the sandy trail, and the wind blew
aside little puffs of dust where the dry dirt was deepest. At no
place was the entire road bare. Grass grew in the middle between
the wheel tracks, worn so deeply in some places as to leave quite
a ridge in the middle. This trail had been in use long before
the Dakota settlers came. It had been a road to market for the
farmers of northern Nebraska for many years.

It was only the fourth day of June, but the sun was beating
down with a midsummer intensity. We all wore hats to shade
our faces. The twins had broad-rimmed sailor hats, anchored
by rubber bands looped under their braids. This was a half-
century before the fad for lying in the sun to get a tan. Thirty
years after this my husband's mother on a late summer visit to
us was to ask me, in deep concern, "Do you think you can get
Elizabeth bleached out in time to start to school?" So we wore
the hats to protect us not only from sunburn, but also from
tanning, a futile gesture for that purpose, however. People of
the prairies always get tanned.

When I went down to Washington University in Saint
Louis, fresh from the prairie country and with no knowledge of
any other habitat, I was aware I looked different from the city
girls. The skins of the girls I saw in Saint Louis were all
delicately pink and white, white from lack of tanning and pink
from rouge and lipstick that I had not yet learned to use. One
of my classmates said to me teasingly, "You must have been out

of doors a lot this summer." It would be a compliment now—
"What a nice tan you have"—but in that day, and from him, it
was a ribbing.

Mother had a black parasol that she tried to use for additional protection from the sun, but the wind was too strong to
make it practicable. The wind seems always to be blowing in a
prairie country. Poets have written of the rippling of prairie
grasses. Rippling is too mild a word. A forceful surging is a
more nearly accurate description. The rippling is only the
minor quavering of the grass blades as they are bent almost
horizontal by the wind. A hunting guide in Wyoming once
told my husband, "If the wind stopped blowing all of a sudden,
them critters would all fall over on their sides."

All of a sudden Fern lurched forward in his seat in front of
us and began yelling, "A pin's sticking me! A pin's sticking me!"

"But there isn't a pin in your blouse anywhere," mother re-
monstrated, but Fern kept on howling, so she leaned over the
seat, loosened the top buttons of his blouse, cupped out his collar in the back, and peered inside. As she did so, a large grasshopper jumped out, lit on Floyd's knee and then went over the
side of the wagon to the ground. Floyd doubled up with laughter, and soon had Fern laughing with him.

The road now descended rather sharply into a hollow, and
we were surprised when Duke and Barney lurched forward with
such alacrity that father had to rein them back rather firmly to
keep them from jolting us and the wagon to pieces with their
burst of speed. At the bottom of the hollow the reason for the
horses' sudden energy was apparent. The road crossed a small
stream. Duke and Barney stretched their necks longingly toward
the water and would have plunged into it, but Father reined
them up sharply at the edge. Then he let Fern hold the reins—
we called them lines--while he and Floyd descended from the
wagon and loosed the checkreins, so the horses could get their
heads down to drink. They stepped forward into the water immediately, and began taking long, pleasurable draughts of it.
They sank their muzzles as deeply as they dared, the current
carrying little eddies of water up to the edge of their nostrils.
Then they would swing their heads sidewise, letting some of the
coolness dribble from their jowls over their hot flanks.

When father was satisfied that they had drunk all they
could hold, he had to speak sharply to them to urge them along,
out of the water.

"Duke! Barney! Giddap now, boys. No more fooling!"

The stream was not more than twenty feet across, and at
the farther edge they stopped again for a few more swallows.

The opposite bank was steeper than the one we had just descended. Duke and Barney seemed to flatten and broaden their powerful bodies in their task of drawing the wagon to the top, while we leaned forward and clung tightly to our seats, a reaction against the fear of slipping backward.

On level ground again, we stopped to fasten the check-reins. Pete, with his mules and load of household goods, was now within easy hailing distance behind us.

"Better give your mules a swig, too," father called to him. Which was apparently what the mules had intended, for they had already started down the decline toward the water at a swift trot, causing mother to turn and watch, apprehensive lest some of our furniture be dislodged.

"How did Duke and Barney know we were coming to water?" Fern wanted to know.

"Oh, animals can smell water," Floyd told him sagely.

"Or maybe they remember it from the trips they made over this road when we were building the house," father added, making it possible for Fern to take or leave his brother's nature lore.

"Will this crick ever be a great big river?" Fern now asked. Fern was usually full of questions.

"It won't be here at all, this fall," father told him. "By the end of August it will be as dry as these wheel tracks."

"I'm thirsty, too," Marie said, wriggling about between mother and me, on the back seat.

"We'll all get a drink when we get to Paxton," father promised.

"You're hot, aren't you?" mother said sympathetically to this smallest member of the family. She loosed the rubber band from under Marie's braids, pushed back her sailor hat, and wiped the moist little face with her handkerchief.

Marjory, the chubbier twin, had been standing between the two seats and leaning forward to watch, round-eyed, as the horses swallowed their large visible gulps of water. Her hat was hanging down her back. Mother set it straight on her head again.

"You must keep your hat on, Margie," mother told her. "I'm afraid we're all going to get as brown as the Indians in this country, if we aren't careful."

"Will we look like the Indians?" Floyd asked, excitedly, looking greatly pleased at the prospect.

"Floyd! You wouldn't want to!" mother exclaimed in horror.

Father turned to look at her with an amused twinkle in his

eyes, but mother's face remained troubled. Here was another piece of the old worry that had been the subject of so many discussions before the final decision had been made, to leave the familiar places in our lives and come to this new country. I, the oldest child, had heard and understood some of these discussions.

"Will it be a good place to bring up the children?" had been much of the burden of mother's concern.

"We'll be doing the bringing up. No reason why we can't do as good a job there as here," had been father's contention.

Although mother had capitulated, she was not convinced. There are so many things about bringing up children that a man does not understand, she thought.

After another half hour father pointed to a group of buildings in the distance. "That's Paxton," he said.

Fern's face fell with disappointment. "But I thought you said we were coming to a town."

"That's a town," father told him; "as big a town as you'll see around here in many a mile."

"It's the first town I've ever seen with only three buildings in it," Fern persisted, solemnly.

"You're not seeing one now," father told him. "There's a blacksmith shop on the other side of that last one you see."

So there was, making four buildings in all—a general store, a saloon, a recreation hall, and the blacksmith shop, not much more than a shed, beside the store. There was a watering trough and pump in front of the store, just beyond a row of hitching posts, where one team hitched to a spring wagon, and two saddle horses were tied. There was a tin cup hanging from a loop of wire fastened to the pump spout. We all got down from the wagon and took turns drinking, while the boys pumped. Pete had been lagging some distance behind us in the past few miles. His mules were getting tired, or maybe balky, father said, and he had been looking back occasionally to make sure Pete was still on the move. Father did not place much dependence upon mules. Pete was close behind us again as we came back to the trail, however. He waved, and called out that he was going along without stopping at Paxton.

"He probably has something with him to drink," father remarked.

"What do you mean?" mother asked fearfully. She did not want our precious belongings in the charge of a drinking man.

"I meant he probably has a water jug," father explained, unconvincingly.

About a quarter of a mile past Paxton, father said with a

new thrill in his voice, "Now we are getting home, this is Tripp County we are in now, our county."

Now our road become wholly an unpredictable trail. It meandered along on the easiest course, avoiding buttes, steep banks and large rocks, unhampered by fences or any other restrictions except those interposed by nature. Shortly after noon we passed a very new homestead. There was a tiny house and barn, unpainted as many of those in Gregory County had been, but in these the wood was still bright and new, unweathered by long exposure to the elements. There was a man out in front, digging a post hole.

"You folks had your dinner?" he called to us. "Better come in. The missus can take care of you."

"Thanks. But we'd better get along," father replied. "Want to get unloaded and straightened out before dark."

"Who was he?" mother asked.

"I don't know," father said. "I never saw him before."

"You never saw him before!" mother exclaimed. "And he would invite all seven of us to dinner?"

Father chuckled. "You'll have to get used to that out here," he said. "You don't have to be acquainted with somebody to invite him to dinner. If he happens along at mealtime, that's all that's necessary."

I could see that there was something very comforting to mother in this incident, and there was to me, too. The thought of this vast new country itself was not at all disturbing to me; on the contrary, I found it exhilarating. Being completely among strangers was the circumstance that had caused me secret little flashes of terror, as I did not meet people easily. Now, in this one triviality, the major part of this feeling was dispelled.

We learned later that the name of this hospitable stranger was George Dall. He had been a street car conductor in Chicago. We became well acquainted with him, his wife Myrtle, and their three children. None of them had any knowledge of rural life, and George knew nothing about farming. He was alert and adaptable, however; he sought and received much advice and tutoring from the seasoned farmers around him, earning their liking and respect, as did his wife and children.

Another house a little farther on was so tiny it was little more than a box, still bright with the raw newness of unfinished lumber. It belonged to a bachelor Frenchman, Henri Mignery where he came from, soon changed to Henry Minnery here.

As we drove farther away from the Gregory County line we were leaving all the old settlements behind us, "old" in the sense of several years. For long stretches no sign of human habitation was in sight. No buildings, no telephone poles, no fences. The only mark of humans was the trail we were following, and that was made by Nebraskans, not Dakotans. Within the year it would look different here. New people were coming in, as we were, to build homes and break the land to a farming civilization. Some were to question the wisdom of this later, when drought, dust storms, and grasshoppers devastated the land in surges. They were to be asking whether it would not have been better to have left the prairies to their natural productiveness without struggling to convert them from grazing lands to orthodox grain farming. The story was told that an old Indian, looking at some of the prairie sod freshly turned over by the breaking plow, shook his head and said, "Wrong side up."

The sun blazed on without a cloud in the sky. Our gallant Duke and Barney began to show signs of fatigue. Their pace became slower, their heads hung a little lower, and they no longer volunteered to surge forward in a mild trot on the downgrades, a motion that shook and rippled their heavy bodies in unison. Patches of sweat darkened their bay and white coats, and the odor of moist horsehair and leather was wafted back to us. This odor was not unpleasant to me as a rule. Now it gave me a pang of homesickness. It smelled like going for a Sunday afternoon drive to Little Grandma's house, in our fine fringe-topped carriage behind the sleek black driving team. On the way we would be thinking what fun it would be to surprise Little Grandma with our visit. But she never failed to say, "I was just thinking you might come today." How we marveled at this prescience of hers! We never guessed that since we were in her thoughts always, it would have been impossible to take her unaware.

We were all tired, tired and hot. "There's nothing to make a shadow," mother said. "If we could just see some shade somewhere, it wouldn't seem quite so hot."

It was years later that I read O. Rolvaag's fine novel, *Giants in the Earth,* about the pioneers in eastern South Dakota in an earlier day. The plaint of his unhappy heroine, Beret, "There's nothing to hide behind!" made me think instantly of my mother. As I read the words, an understanding of mother's true feeling burst upon me for the first time. It was not the heat that oppressed her most. This was only the first week in June; it would be much hotter in the next two months, and we would endure it. Not the heat, but the vast unshelteredness all about us, the same thing that troubled Beret.

There was much similarity between mother and Beret, I realized as I read. They shared many of the same fears. Mother's fears, however, never weighted her into anything comparable to Beret's depressions. Whether or not she was saved from this by a sufficiently supporting factor in her environment might be a matter of dispute, but I believe she was, and that this saving support was my father. She was so woefully dependent upon him, and at the same time had such complete trust in him, that she could never have felt lost while he was by her side. She thought of him as an indestructible anchor to which she was firmly tethered.

We came to a place where a barbed wire fence, the first fence we had seen in Tripp County, crossed our trail. There was no gate. Father and Floyd got down from the wagon, lifted the wires off their fastenings on the posts, pulled them down to the ground and stood on them, while Duke and Barney stepped carefully across at father's command, with Fern proudly holding the lines.

"My, some settler must have fenced in a lot of land for himself," mother commented, following with her eyes the line of fence posts that continued on out of sight over a distant slope.

"It isn't a settler's fence at all," father explained. "It was put up by the cattlemen, for their range cattle. This fellow Laird's got a six-mile square fenced. Some of his cattle are still running here."

"There will be a gate in the fence around our place, won't there?" Fern wanted to know.

Father laughed. "Our place doesn't have any fence around it yet, at all," he said.

"What does it have around it?" Fern pressed, soberly.

"Nothing," father said.

"Then how do we know where it is and where it isn't?"

"It has been surveyed," father explained, "and there is a little pile of rocks at each corner. When we have time, we'll build a fence to each of those corners."

Fern lapsed into silence and apparent discouragement. And without committing myself by speech, I was suddenly as disheartened as he. I looked around me. We had all been trying to envision what our place would look like. It must be just a spot.

Our trail had meandered but had kept a persistent westerly course. Now it turned sharply south. A red barn stood at this turn, the only painted barn we had seen. The settlers were living in it while they were building their house.

Each of us was eager to be the first to identify our house. Father had said he would not point it out to us; we must recognize it from his own rather meager description. The land was more rolling now, and as we came over each new rise we would peer ahead along the trail for the small unpainted house and barn that would be different from the others only because it was ours.

At the top of a long hill, we had a far-reaching vista into the valley before us. About halfway between the low lying hills on either side was some kind of habitation.

"Maybe that's it!" the boys called out excitedly, in unison.

"No, it couldn't be," mother told them. "That house has an ell. Ours is built in just one straight length."

Father refused to comment one way or the other.

As we came closer, however, we saw that what had looked like an ell was really the barn, which was between us and the house, and even father could remain noncommittal no longer. He admitted that this was our new home.

The house was a small two-room shack, quite typical of the first homes built in the Rosebud Country. Its dimensions were sixteen by twenty-four feet. When I was married, the first house we lived in had a living room exactly that size. I used to look at it and wonder how seven people could have lived in that restricted space. The barn was large enough to accommodate two teams of horses. The newness of it all was rather zestful, and at the same time rather terrifying. No fence, no garden spot, no trees, no permanent well dug. We procured water from a hole about three feet deep, which Father had dug in a low spot near a pond. The usual sources of water contamination were not to be feared here. The drainage into that pond had probably never washed over even the footprint of another human being.

It was now midafternoon, and we were all hungry. Father set a small gasoline stove on the ground beside the house, and lifted a box of dishes and cooking utensils, and a bag of groceries down from the wagon, so that mother might prepare dinner. Then he and Pete unhitched the horses and mules, watered them and turned them out to eat grass, while they unloaded our furnishings and set them in the house.

In about an hour mother had unpacked the requisite utensils and food, and with my dubious help had dinner prepared. There was coffee, bacon, canned corn, potatoes boiled with their skins on, store cookies and bakery bread, "punky, no-good stuff" father always characterized the latter. There was Karo corn syrup for our bread, and we poured a little bacon fat on our potatoes. Everything tasted fine.

It seems now that it must have been quite a task, but before Pete and his mules left for their own place, about dusk, all our goods had been unloaded and set inside the house. Beds had been set up, and enough bedding unpacked to accommodate us all for the night. We were tired, and shortly after dark we were all in bed asleep.

The boys slept on a folding bed beside the kitchen window, which as yet had no screen. In the night Fern wakened us all with a scream of terror, and mother and father ran to him to see what was the matter. Some of the wild range cattle had come up to investigate this puzzling intrusion on their grazing land, and one of the more venturesome steers had put his head through the window and sniffed noisily in Fern's face. Fern's scream had been all that was needed to drive them away. They were in as much of a panic as Fern was. We could hear the whole herd galloping away in the distance.

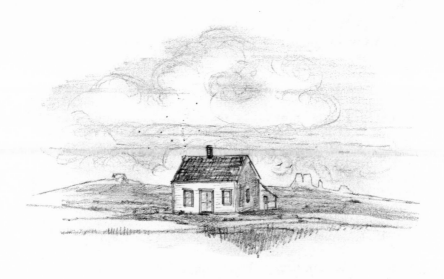

5 / DAYS OF SERENITY

QUIETUDE is a feature of the virgin prairie difficult to recall accurately, impossible to describe. No words embellish it, as no words embellish peace, or contentment. There are many adjectives for their disruptive antagonists, but each of these three abstract nouns must stand alone in its crystalline purity. We, with our chatterings and bustlings about, were interlopers in a vast realm of silence. We were almost the only noisemakers. The few exceptions were the occasional thunderstorms, the wind, a flock of south-flying geese in the fall, the howl of a coyote at dusk, the miniscule insect sounds in the grass. If we walked near a pond in the evening we might hear the croaking of frogs, perhaps a splash or two as some of them jumped into the water to escape these human invaders, the like of which they had never seen before.

In the summertime the stillness inside the house would be broken by daylight, with father's peremptory, "Time to get up!" or mother's more gentle, "Breakfast is nearly ready, boys," and then a pat on my shoulder and a whispered summons to come and set the table—whispered to avoid waking the twins sleeping beside me, the ubiquitous twins, four years old, whom the rest of us would have been glad to permit to sleep half the morning. But they rarely failed to tumble sleepily out of bed after me, and by the time I had the table set would be dressed and sitting on the boys' bed in the kitchen, where the family activity was, chattering to their dolls.

I envied them their childish determination to be alert participants in the doings of the day. The dragging process of my own dressing would have been accomplished with no eagerness and with many longing looks at the rumpled bed, where it would have seemed the most heavenly luxury to have slept for another hour. I was prodded out of the temptation to lie down again, just for a minute, by the inexorable sounds from the kitchen reminding me that the activities of the day were on the march and that I must get into step—the rattling of the stove lids that accompanied the kindling of the fire, the sound of water being poured from the dipper into the tin wash basin for hasty morning face washings, the grating sound of skillets and pans being moved across the top of the stove telling me that breakfast was already well under way.

A plains breakfast was a meal, one of the day's three, perhaps less varied than the other two but just as calorific. There would be oatmeal, ham or bacon, eggs, slices from the enormous loaves of mother's bread which we spread with corn syrup or sorghum or whatever preserve or jelly was at hand, and always potatoes. Sometimes the potatoes were "fresh fried" but these were an emergency dish, not a first choice. Peeling, slicing, and frying the raw potatoes took much longer to prepare than what came to be called later "hashed browns," which we always tried to have available. These were prepared by chopping the boiled potatoes left over from supper the night before and frying them in drippings. We did the chopping with an empty baking powder can which had a sharp-edged top. The process took only a few minutes. Sometimes we had hot baking powder biscuits, but these, too, were apt to be an emergency treat, provided when we had run out of bread. There was no limit to the variety of other foods that might appear on our breakfast table at various times. Availability was the only requisite. Nothing was ruled out because it was inappropriate for breakfast. If it was good to eat, it was as good at breakfast as at any other meal. Pie left over from last night's supper, for example, would be finished off by the boys at breakfast with gusto.

Father and the boys usually had the farm chores done before breakfast. With the meal over, they hurried out to the major part of the farm work. Father always hurried; he never moved deliberately, seeming always to have the routine of his day's activities fixed like a map in his mind, probably sketched there before he went to sleep the night before, so that there was no necessity for wasteful contemplation during working hours.

The first necessity for the new settlers was housing for family and animals, although we seldom referred to these first homes as houses. We called them "claim shacks," with a sort of braggadocio. We knew they were nothing grand, hardly respectable, but what the heck. We were all in the same boat, on a wonderful ship of pioneering and exploration which would carry us to wealth or fame or discovery, according to the form of our fantasies.

Our tiny claim shack was divided into two rooms, a bedroom and the slightly larger room that was used for everything else, including a bedroom for the two boys. We achieved some privacy in the bedroom by dividing it in half with a cloth curtain strung on a wire. Boxes under the beds provided storage. Keeping things sorted out and in some useful order was one of the main problems of housekeeping.

The second necessity, almost as important as the housing, was getting some land under cultivation as quickly as possible to provide food for both family and animals. Father had done a token amount of plowing which had been planted to corn and potatoes when he came up in the spring to build the house and barn, thus insuring some food for us and the horses. There was a beneficence connected with a crop of "sod corn" which was never repeated later. It did not need to be plowed. It could not be plowed, in fact, being interwoven with a network of grass roots which had not yet disintegrated. Also, this newly turned sod had not yet been defiled with weed seeds, so that weeds were no problem. Given a year, however, the weeds would flourish and offer constant battle to the crops. Good potatoes could be grown on new sod, but they had one peculiarity. The ones that developed between the layer of overturned sod and the earth beneath would be flattened on two sides as though they had been pressed between two boards.

The very earliest breaking of the prairie, done by every homesteader, was really an adjunct to his house building, not for crop purposes at all. This was the plowing of several furrows completely around his buildings, as a fire guard. This was apt to be done as soon as the lumber was unloaded, before the building was actually started. Prairie fires were a constant menace, and they were not an imaginary one, by any means. Often at night we saw their ominous glow on the horizon. The interposition of a strip of bare earth between a settler's holdings and the sweeping flames was an effective protection.

Being the oldest, and a girl, my job was naturally mother's helper. With our belongings unpacked and stowed away as compactly as possible, gardening was next on our priority list.

"My, it's late to be getting a garden in," mother fretted. "A lot of vegetables are apt to be caught by frost. They won't have time to mature before fall."

The tenth of April had always been garden planting time

on mother's calendar, and here it was the end of the first week in June. Nevertheless, we would do the best we could. With all her worry, this garden planting afforded mother much amusement. All we had to do was to prod little holes into the sod and drop the seeds in. Trenches could not be marked in rows with a hoe as in previously tilled ground, because, again, of those fine little grass roots that enmeshed the soil. Nor did any hoeing need to be done, a circumstance to make any gardener jubilant. I think mother never quite trusted this bizarre form of gardening until she saw the little green shoots appearing, promptly as in any oldtime garden. This first year there were several nice June rains to nourish our optimism.

Our long forenoons were ample time for the major housework chores and gardening, except on bread baking days. Making bread with the old-fashioned yeast was a slow process. Started the evening before, it always encroached on most of the next afternoon. But what a superb product mother always turned out! A compliment that delighted and amused her was a dictum agreed upon by the twins, "Mother's bread is as light and puffy as anybody else's angel food."

All this left several afternoons a week free for explorations in this new land, which we liked to think no one else knew about except us. While father spent the afternoon plowing, mother, the boys, the twins, and I took long walks. Usually we went south or west. We had driven into Tripp County from the north and east, so we had seen that area once. The unknown was more thrilling. No fences, no roads, only occasional paths worn by the range cattle in their trek to ponds or streams for water. There was one house in sight south of us, about the age of ours, and the owner had not yet arrived to take up her occupancy. She was a school teacher, we had heard, from the eastern part of the state, and her father, who had had homesteading experience in his own youth, would be staying most of the required fourteen months with her.

Mother always carried a long stick on these walks, perhaps a hoe or a rake, for fear of ratlesnakes. Not that she ever intended to kill one. She used the stick to part any long grasses before we walked through them, just in case one of these dread reptiles should be lurking there. A great many rattlesnakes did live in our neighborhood, but experience taught us that they were never found in these lush areas of tall grass, only in the more barren, rocky, sunny spots such as occurred higher on the buttes. We learned, too, that the story of rattlesnakes living in prairie dog towns was no myth, as we had thought. There was a prairie dog town across the road from our house, and to mother's continuing alarm, the boys would make projects of going over to the prairie dog town to kill rattlesnakes. The weapons they used were some beer bottles left by the men who had helped father build the house. (There was no beer ever in our household.) When mother protested against this type of hunting which she considered so hazardous, as it doubtless was, the boys would reply, innocently, "Well, would you rather we left the rattlesnakes alive? They are awful close to our house."

The rattlesnake was one species of wildlife that no one ever campaigned to preserve, so far as I am aware. Total extinction was the aim of the settlers. Seeing a rattlesnake and letting it live was a crime against our society. They were considered very easy to kill. One afternoon when Fern and I were riding horseback along the side of a butte west of our claim, we heard the ominous whirring warning that was unmistakable, once heard. Horses recognized it as easily as people. We thought at first that we could not possibly kill this snake, having no weapon of any kind. There are never any sticks to be picked up on the prairie. Sometimes rocks are lying about but none were here. We were so reluctant to flout the law of the settlers about leaving a rattler alive that Fern finally took the bridle off his horse and slapped the reptile to death with the reins. The horse stood quietly by until its bridle was replaced, apparently cooperating consciously in this worthy deed. I could not estimate how many rattlers the boys killed. I know that for years they had a Mason fruit jar full of the rattles they had preserved. This trophy collection was very repugnant to mother, and I think she finally buried it.

The Dakota solitudes were a nurturing background for meditation, and I thought deeply about many things, among them about those rattlesnakes. They were thoughts I dared not confide to anyone. Notwithstanding respect for justice, few people feel warmth toward a lawyer who defends a murderer. No one in the prairie country would have conceded that a rattlesnake has any good qualities, and a protagonist for such a creature would have had his sanity doubted. Nevertheless, comparisons favorable to the rattlesnake kept recurring to me. What other wild creature gave its enemies warning in such a sporting manner?

Thus when I reached the verse-writing stage that so many introspective young people go through, it was probably only natural that the rattlesnake should be one of the subjects of my inspiration; should be, in fact, the subject of the only sonnet I ever wrote. Shades of Elizabeth Barrett Browning! Sonnets are supposed to be written about love! I had a guilty sense of desecration as I labored over my lines.

The only awareness of any other member of the serpent group, besides occasional harmless garter snakes, that had been impressed upon me was by way of a picture in the family Bible showing a loathsome coil of python proportions, embodiment of deceit, evil, and treachery, draped in and about a tree in the Garden of Eden, offering the first taste of sin to the innocent Eve. The first half of my sonnet, therefore, depicted the abhorrent character of the biblical serpent, and closed with this brief for the comparative virtues of the rattlesnake.

> The rattler's blow
> Strikes in defense of his own solitude.
> No ambush hides his spotted length; he lies
> Brazenly on the barren rock; and, scorning
> Trickery and the masked intent, he eyes
> With frank malevolence the one who passes,
> Unbidden, through his lair in sunburned grasses,
> Dry and brittle as his deadly warning.

I like to believe that my sonnet's uniqueness compensated for any lack of poetic virtue. It was not only the only sonnet I ever wrote, but is also, so far as I know, the only sonnet anyone has ever written on that subject.

In a dry country, water is a necessity not taken for granted. It is a considered, hoped for beneficence, and the very sight of it is refreshing. We were about as far from a seacoast as it is possible to get. The Missouri River, seen on the map, appears to be no great distance, but with our methods of travel it was inaccessible to us except on a major journey. Our nearest river, the Keya Paha, was as small a stream as is ever designated by name on a map, and we saw that only two or three times in a year. Occasional other creeks had names locally, but they were apt to be dried up by late summer, to come alive again only with the thawing of next winter's snow, followed by spring rains.

Making provision for an adequate water supply for family and livestock cost father some hard labor this first summer. Our temporary well was about three feet deep, in a low spot beside a pond. We drew up the water in a galvanized pail by an attached rope. This water always had an oily sheen on the surface, especially noticeable in coffee, which did not affect the taste, however. We used to wonder, vaguely, about the possibility of oil deposits under the land, but never gave any serious thought to it. The settlers here were interested in farming, not in oil wells. This shallow well, we knew, could be only a summer makeshift. In the winter the water would be frozen, and often the entire site buried in snow. One of the jobs that had to be done before winter was the digging of a permanent well, deep enough so that the water would not freeze, to which a hand pump could be attached, thus insuring us a year-round water supply.

After days of back-breaking digging by hand, with a spade, with no underground stream of water encountered, father was forced to fill the dirt in the hole again and to repeat the whole process at the opposite corner of our claim. Here he did strike water at a depth he considered within reason, and after the water rose steadily, promising to make a continuing reservoir of supply, he installed a pump. Thus we were assured of all the water we would need, but it was a half-mile away! Nothing to do now but move the house and barn to a new location, near the well, which, with the help of other settlers and their teams, was done. This was the most discouraging episode in our first year, not only because of the added work involved, but because the house suffered damage in the process. Some of the plaster was cracked, and patches of it fell off the bedroom walls which was distressful enough at the time, but was to become much more so later.

To people in a plains country, water is something more than a necessity. Water is beautiful, to be looked at with delight, wherever found. In our wanderings about the countryside, the little ponds in the vicinity attracted us more strongly than any other feature. They were the places we looked for, and returned to, again and again.

"Where shall we go today?" was a question apt to draw such replies as, "It's hot this afternoon; let's just go down to the first pond." Or, "Let's go clear down to the big pond where we saw so many fish." Or, "I'd like to walk over that row of buttes; there might be some ponds below them, or maybe a creek."

We usually took off our shoes and stockings and waded for a while in the shallow edges of any pond we came to. In the evenings after a hot afternoon our entire family might go bathing in the nearest pond. Finding fish in some of the larger ponds was an ecstatic discovery. There was no need for guessing whether or not there might be fish. We could see them darting about in the clear water as plainly as if they had been in a glass bowl—sunfish, redhorse, suckers, and catfish. The first time we saw them, the boys could hardly wait to dash home and get their fishing tackle.

"Are you sure we brought any fishhooks and lines with us?" mother asked dubiously.

Floyd was certain we had. He had packed them in a special box of his own, and he knew just where to find it. He did find it promptly, and he and Fern began making enthusiastic plans to go fishing in the morning.

"What will you use for poles?" mother asked. "You can't find any nice straight tree branches here, or any other kind of branches."

Floyd's face fell, and he was speechless. Fern was at the point of tears. He stamped his foot and exclaimed, "I never saw such a rotten country! Not a tree in it anywhere!"

Father had been splashing his face and hands in the wash basin just outside the kitchen door, preparatory to coming in to supper. While combing his hair he overheard Fern's outburst, and peered in through the screen to ask, "What do you mean, no trees in this country? You haven't looked over all our claim yet. You go up over that hill just east of the barn, and down the other side, and you'll see some trees."

Both boys looked the incredulity they dared not express in words. No one ever questioned a statement of father's. After this momentary hesitation, they accepted it as truth, as a good Christian accepts a miracle, believed though not understood. They wanted to go, right now, to see the trees, the existence of which they no longer doubted.

Mother, however, interposed objections. "It's suppertime," she said, "and getting dark. We wouldn't be able to see anything by the time we got there. We'll all go in the morning."

The next morning, after household chores were done, all of us except father trooped up the hill back of the barn and down the steep slope on the other side. From the top of the hill we could see some density of the greenery, something more than the prairie grass. This spot would be the northeast corner of our claim, father had said. Here, indeed, were the trees father had promised, a clump of willows hardly more than bushes, and three other trees not much taller than a man, with clusters of green fruit on them.

"Choke cherries!" mother exclaimed with pleasure. "I've heard people say they grew here."

She restrained the boys in their eagerness to break off some of the largest branches, urging them to choose ones that had the least fruit on them. Fern had already bitten into one of the cherries, and spit it out.

"They're no good!" he said, making a wry face. "They make my mouth feel all puckered."

"They don't do that so much when they're ripe," mother told him, "but they always do have a little of that effect. That's where they get the name 'choke' cherries."

At the base of the willows was a creek bed, with the merest trickle of water in it. This was Lute's Creek, which father had said cut through this corner of our claim. Having a creek on our own land seemed like a bonus to us, but father did not regard it so. He said it was no good for anything, and ruined that part of the claim for farming.

In spite of mother's restrictions, the boys were able to find a branch apiece that would do as a fishing pole, and we all went fishing that afternoon. It was a happy and successful trip. We came home with six little sunfish and several suckers, which, beheaded, scaled and eviscerated, then rolled in cornmeal and fried, made a succulent if not very full platter of food for supper. We had fished before, in the Brushy and Raccoon Rivers in Iowa, but this kind of fishing was different. There was no need for a bobbing cork to tell us when we had a bite. The water was so clear we could see every move the fish made. This fishing excursion was repeated many times during the rest of the summer.

As we wandered farther and farther from home in our walks about the countryside, mother gradually lost her timidity, having met no rattlers or other hazards, except an occasional indiscreet contact with a cactus plant. We knew better than to grasp, or even to touch, one of these plants, but sometimes they would be unseen beside a prairie flower we stooped to pick. They had sharp spiny projections all over them, which in turn, were covered with microscopic barbs, like fishhooks. Once they had penetrated the flesh they could not be pulled out cleanly. The tissue around them had to soften, or even suppurate, before they were loosed. On one of our walks I was wearing a pair of shoes so nearly worn out that they were thin-soled, and one of these cruel cactus spines, stepped upon inadvertently, went through my shoe into the sole of my foot. For two weeks or more my foot was so sore I could not take a flat step, but had to walk with my foot twisted protectively.

Wildflowers were everywhere. None of us knew anything about botany, and we made up our own names for them. They grew in such masses that entire hillsides would be tinted with the color of their blooms—pink, blue, yellow, lavender. What we called wild sweet peas were most common. Our favorite variety for bouquets had bell-shaped lavender blossoms distributed along tall stalks; we called these dream flowers. At first we brought handfuls of flowers home from every walk we took, and put them in jars and jelly glasses in the house, but we found we took little enjoyment in looking at them there. The bouquets were mostly in the way in our crowded quarters, and the flowers not so beautiful as they were in their own natural beds on the hillsides. "They belong out there where they grew," mother said. "Putting them in vases is like trying to bring a piece of the rainbow into the house.

We suffered a bad fright one day, probably needlessly. We had walked over the range of buttes to the west of us, and came suddenly upon a herd of range cattle. We had always been told that one could never get close to these wild cattle, that they would always run from human beings. These, however, probably as startled as we were, merely stopped grazing, stood still and gazed at us. Then several of the ones nearest us started walking forward, cautiously, and the entire herd followed.

Instinctively we turned about, but Floyd warned, out of the knowledge of some wild animal stories he had read, "If we run, they'll chase us!" So we limited our pace to a swift walk, with many fearful backward glances.

"Are they trying to surround us?" mother asked, breathlessly, out of some wild animal lore of her own. "Oh, if there was just a fence for us to crawl under!"

The cattle continued to follow us back over the line of buttes. Coming down the other side, however, some of them stopped to snatch a few mouthfuls of grass, and soon the entire herd was grazing again, paying no more attention to us. We continued on home, our zest for adventuring having petered out for that day. Father tended to pooh-pooh the idea that we had been in danger, but not with complete conviction. It was just curiosity that made them follow us, he said, but it was better to avoid getting that close to them. If something happened to frighten them they could stampede and trample us into the ground.

In mother's opinion, the most rewarding, in a practical way, of any exploring walk we took that first June, was one straight south of our claim. It was an especially beautiful day, neither very windy nor very hot, so we walked on and on, with little regard for distance. We came to another creek which we learned later was one of the meanderings of the same Lute's Creek that crossed our claim. On its banks was a cluster of wild gooseberry bushes, loaded with berries in their prime for picking. Gooseberries were a familiar fruit to us, well liked by us all, with our rugged, youthful tastes. (A self-educated gourmet I met in my later years, in whom I attempted to inculcate an appreciation of this fruit, gave as his firm opinion that it is not possible to get enough sugar into a gooseberry pie to make it edible.)

We started picking them immediately, but our harvesting

was hampered by a lack of containers. Floyd's hat and mother's apron were the only receptacles we had. When we came back the next afternoon, we were better prepared, with a flour sack and several pails. But we overstepped ourselves again. With all of us working through most of the afternoon, we had more berries than we thought we could carry that long distance home. So we poured all the berries into the flour sack, tied a knot in the end, stowed it under one of the bushes, and walked home empty-handed. That evening, after supper, father broke his rule about making farm horses work after their day in the field was done. He let Floyd and me ride Duke and Barney down to get the gooseberries. We rode bareback, as we had not yet acquired any saddles. Floyd, being more acrobatic than I, jumped down from his horse and boosted the sack of berries onto Duke's back, in front of me. Tired as they were, the horses were impatient to get back home again, and even broke into a trot going up the steep side of a gully. With the jolting motion, my ineptness as a horsewoman, the sleek surface of Duke's broad back, and the weight of the berries in front of me, the berries and I slid backward to the ground over Duke's tail. Duke remained unperturbed, and took the occasion to nibble some mouthfuls of grass, while Floyd boosted both his burdens back into place.

We made almost daily berry-picking trips after that, as long as the crop lasted. The industry which the boys and I showed in this job had a pecuniary motive. It was a way we had earned most of our spending money for the Fourth of July in the past several years. Mother paid us five cents a quart, and an extra penny for stemming them after we got home, which was quite lucrative by our standards.

6 | DAKOTA FOURTH

"WILL DAKOTA have a Fourth of July?" Fern asked one day late in June. We all laughed but it was not really a silly question. The Fourth of July was not a date to us. It was a festival. The glorious Fourth! Never was an adjective more aptly applied! It rated higher than birthdays, Valentine's Day, or last day of school, in importance. In some respects it was more exciting than Christmas, being noisier and more raucous and unrestrained.

The holiday had been on our minds a great deal recently, mostly with foreboding. With all the optimism we could muster, it was difficult to imagine a Fourth of July celebration, as we had known them, on these prairies. Then one day father came home from Paxton with a twinkle in his eye and a large, colored poster in his hand. The poster announced that Dallas would be celebrating the Fourth in a big way, with a three-day festival, packed with all the excitement-arousing events ever staged for such an occasion. There would be bands, speeches, fireworks, a merry-go-round, parades, athletic contests, and a multitude of concessions vending the customary attractions in the way of edibles, shooting galleries and side shows. When father topped this exciting announcement by the statement that he had already agreed that we should all go to spend' the entire three days, it was almost more than we could believe. He had talked to the Dalls and the Evanses, who were taking tents in which we could sleep and do our own cooking. They would go to Dallas early on the morning of the Fourth and have the tents pitched on their chosen spot, the schoolhouse yard, by the time we arrived. We lived farther away, and could hardly hope to get there ahead of the crowds.

This was the most irresponsible and reckless binge I ever knew my parents to embark upon. Here we were, barely getting settled in a new pioneer home, with all the labor ahead of us that would be necessary to fortify us against the coming winter, setting out on a profitless three-day carnival! Seemingly profitless, I should say. There must have been immeasurable benefits from this never-to-be-repeated, carefree time of relaxation and enjoyment that bolstered them in many times of stress ahead. This was the one time in their lives it could have been done, before the claim was stocked with all the responsibilities a farmer of that day took upon himself; an invigorating breath before the final plunge into the risks and hazards and the merciless toil involved in making productive farmland out of an inscrutable prairie. We did have an extra team of horses by this

48

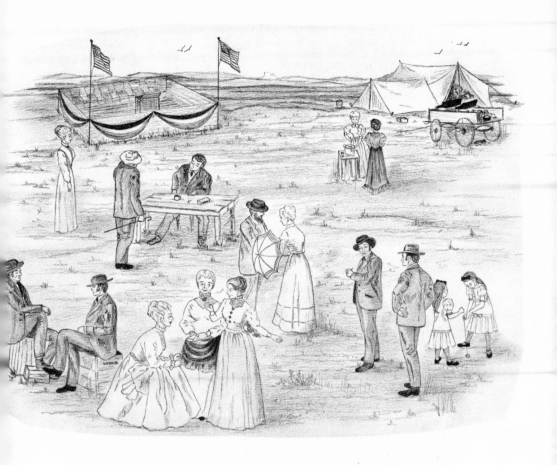

time, but no chickens, cows, or pigs. They would be added in the fall, and they were the kind of stock that needed meticulous daily attention. The horses we left at home could be put to pasture to forage their own food and water.

We were up even earlier than usual on the morning of the Fourth, and ready to start a little after seven. We drove the new team of sorrels, Nell and Gypsy, who were lighter than Duke and Barney, and capable of making better time on the road. Another factor that lightened our transportation was a secondhand, two-seated spring wagon father had bought at a sale in Gregory County the week before. With its seven passengers, some extra clothing, bedding, food baskets, and oats for the horses, it was filled to capacity.

The sky was cloudless, the wind had not yet risen, and the sun was only a benign, basking warmth, still far short of its midday intensity. Mother opened her parasol and tilted it toward the east, more as a dutiful gesture against tanning than as a protection from the heat. Even the horses seemed to be imbued with the holiday spirit. They arched their necks and would have kept their pace at a rapid trot, except for father's restraining hand on the reins.

"You've got a long way to go yet, my pretties," father told them.

"Nell and Gypsy like to go to the Fourth, too, don't they?" Marjory commented.

"Aw, they don't know where we're going!" Fern scoffed.

"I bet they do!" both twins chimed in unison, whereupon to circumvent dissension, mother diverted everyone's attention to the Smith house we were passing. This was the family that was living in the barn until they had the house built. Now the house was nearly finished, an imposing one for this country, being the only one for miles around that had two stories.

As the sun rose higher, a shimmering heat haze rose in the distance. The scent of the prairie grasses was in our nostrils, faintly sharp and faintly bitter, like an inhaled tonic. Several times we heard a meadowlark, and craned our necks for a sight of the singer, but he kept himself hidden. The twins became drowsy and leaned their heads against mother and me for fitful naps.

"Now we're almost there, aren't we?" Fern asked when we came to Paxton.

"Not halfway yet," Floyd told him, cruelly, out of his older brother wisdom.

Mother and father hoped to arrive in time to hear the program in the park. The rest of us just wanted to get there. After another hour, Nell and Gypsy had lost some of their exuberance. They no longer persisted in a trot, but would have settled for a steady walk except for father's occasional verbal prodding, accompanied by slaps of the reins, "Giddap, Gyp, Nell! Let's not go to sleep!"

At last, on the cemetery hill, we could see Dallas. The boys bounced up and down in their seats, and their excited talk wakened the twins. We all began straining our eyes and our ears for the first intimations of the delights ahead of us. Mother, however, had seemed preoccupied for a few minutes. Finally she leaned forward and touched father on the shoulder.

"Isn't that an automobile coming over there on the Gregory road?" she asked.

"Well, I shouldn't be surprised," father replied calmly, after looking sharply in the direction she indicated. "There's several got them now, in Dallas and Gregory both."

We all watched the approaching cloud of dust intently.

"It is an auto! It is an auto!" Floyd shouted. "A team couldn't be coming that fast!"

Mother looked at him with tolerant reproof. Floyd was just the one to welcome excitement, even if it meant danger to us all.

"My, I wish we'd drove Duke and Barney," she said, anxiously. "It's a safer thing to do when we know we might meet automobiles. Gyp gets so awfully scared."

Father defended himself. "A heavy work team can't stand road trips like this; it takes too much flesh off them. There's nothing to get excited about."

The approaching vehicle was an automobile, right enough; a shiny new red one.

"It might be Doc Jorgensen," father observed. "They say he got one lately."

The road was cut down somewhat through the cemetery hill, so that there was a steep bank arising on either side. Father drove close to the right bank, and stopped the team. Then he handed the lines to Fern, and he and Floyd got out and stood at the mares' heads, holding them firmly by the bridles, close to the bits.

"Oh, I don't think any of us had better stay in, do you?" mother asked, with an alarm that communicated itself to all of us, even to father.

The car was quite close by this time. Its machinery was plainly audible, and Gypsy was beginning to prance about. Father considered for a moment, then took the lines from Fern and wrapped them around the handle of the buggy whip, and Fern and the rest of us got out and clambered up the bank, father and Floyd retaining their hold on the horses' bridles.

The driver of the car, whoever he was, was a considerate gentleman. He slowed down from his speed of twenty miles an hour, and made as wide a detour as possible as he passed us. Nell was fairly stolid as to temperament, but Gypsy was a jumpy one indeed. Her fright was pitiable to see. She cowered, wild-eyed, as far from the apparition as possible, shaking in every muscle. I heard mother catch her breath several times as she watched. If she should fall against that wagon tongue and break it! But Gypsy made no effort to bolt, or to break from father's restraining hand. It was all over in a few moments—that was one good thing about the episode—and we all resumed our places. Poor Gypsy's coat was wet with sweat, and she started forward with a lurch at father's signal, eager to be gone as quickly as possible from the site of her terror.

Now we were practically there; the rest of the trip was only a drawing out of the pleasure of arriving. We saw other vehicles on the way; some ahead of us and some on the two crossroads between us and Dallas. There were spring wagons like ours, some lumber wagons filled with celebrators, several shiny-top buggies, each containing a fellow and his girl. The horses hitched to these latter vehicles had their harness decorated with little flags and with red, white, and blue pompons, and we gazed after them admiringly.

All Dallas was aflutter with flags and bunting, and soon the delightful cacophony associated with the Fourth became audible—the staccato pop of firecrackers, the rhythmic squawk of the merry-go-round, the excited voices of children, the dying wail of deflated balloons, shouts of hawkers, and, covering it all with lively overtones, the band playing "Yankee Doodle."

"That's my favorite tune!" Fern said, ecstatically. Floyd and I joined in the parental laughter, but not very heartily. We were too nearly of the same opinion ourselves.

At the post office corner a man stepped out from the crowd and hailed us. It was George Dall. "The tents are set up," he said, "down in the schoolhouse yard, the best spot in town. Myrtie and Rachel are there waiting for you."

Rachel was John Evans's wife. The two women were giving a few last minute touches to the arrangements in the tents. They greeted us warmly, their voices infused with the pervading excitement. The two Evans boys and the three Dall children had gone down town where the crowds and the noise were. Father and Floyd unhitched the horses, gave them water and hay, and tethered them to the back of the spring wagon, while the women helped mother and me unload and arrange our camping supplies.

"We'll be in time for the program if we get right down to the park," father said, looking at his watch. The boys had already disappeared. The rest of us walked the three blocks to the park, a grassy plot bordered with saplings in varying states of vigor, several of them already dead. A bandstand stood in the center, and seats had been improvised from planks borrowed from the lumber store to accommodate the holiday crowds.

The band had returned from downtown, and were reassembling on the bandstand, tuning their instruments. Two girls I knew slightly were talking to the drummer. I could hardly imagine being on speaking terms with one of those gorgeously uniformed figures. In a few moments, three men took their places beside the speaker's rostrum; the congressman from Burke who was to give the address, the mayor who would introduce him, and Chief Yellow Jacket, by far the most colorful of the three, who was usually given a seat of honor and introduced at any of these public functions. It was meant, and accepted, as a friendly gesture, yet there was something painful in it, too; a once important ruling figure thus made a puppet in the entertainments of his conquerors.

It was anything but a quiet place for a speech. Babies were getting fussy for their dinners. Mothers were shushing little ones who were playing with squawkers, and were continually being tempted to blow them just a little. Other children were hopping about in great glee over the empty planks in the back. And in the outskirts, all about, the rest of the celebration proceeded unabated. But no one minded not being able to hear much of what was being said. It was the spirit, the flavor of the thing that mattered, and the speaker was applauded frequently and vociferously as the summits of his oratory reached us in the familiar ringing words and phrases—"our glorious country," "freedom and equality," "our righteous forefathers," "land of liberty." They made delicious little thrills run all over me, and I believed them all.

After the singing of "America" the crowd dispersed rapidly. It was noon, and Fourth of July dinner was one of the important dinners of the year. Our food baskets had already been lifted out of the wagons into the tents, and the men stood about in a helpless sort of impatience while the women set out the food. But the women took their time; there were certain amenities to be observed.

"Now I brought a big tablecloth," Mrs. Evans volunteered, "maybe it will do for everybody."

"But that's a linen one," Mrs. Dall objected, "and a lot of work to do up. I brought one we use just for picnics. It's easy to iron."

"But I want to use mine," Mrs. Evans persisted. "It gets mussy lying in the drawer so long without being done up."

"Why don't you just get out our cloth and put it down?" father said in an undertone to mother, his impatience prodding him into interfering with what was strictly women's business.

So mother put our cloth down without more ado. It was a picnic cloth, too, unused since we had left Iowa. It had a patch on one corner where a pup had chewed it as it hung on the clothesline. Mrs. Dall followed mother's example, and the stage was set for dinner.

There had been no prearrangement as to menu. Each family had brought enough for a complete dinner. Fried chicken was the traditional choice of farm people as the main item on the Fourth of July menu. Chickens large enough to fry, new potatoes and garden peas by the Fourth, were marks of the up-and-coming householder. Here in this new country, however, temporary lapses from the old traditions were excusable. Today, Mrs. Evans was the only one who had brought chicken, and she had had only two of them she considered large enough to fry. We had brought ham, and George Dall had been to the butcher shop after they arrived in Dallas, and bought a generous package of luncheon meat. After the serving started and Mrs. Evans began to fret about the possibility that her chicken would not reach around the crowd, we were relieved to note that most of the children preferred the minced ham and bologna, which were much more of a novelty to them than either the chicken or baked ham.

Arrayed with the meats, against the onslaught of hearty appetites, were baked beans, jams and jellies, homemade bread, beet and cucumber pickles, pies, cakes, and filled cookies. There were eggs, also; some plain hard-boiled and some deviled, the halves put together again neatly with toothpicks. One of the women had fixed her eggs in a fancy manner of her own. After boiling them she had removed the shells and dyed the whites a lovely cerise color in beet juice. I thought Father shuddered slightly as he passed these by. Our drink was lemonade. Each housewife had brought a quantity of sweetened lemon juice in a fruit jar, and Mrs. Dall had borrowed a large stone crock from a friend who worked in a restaurant, to mix it in.

Mothers filled plates for the younger children first. There wasn't room for them around the main picnic spread, so they sat back a little way, on a blanket. No one had napkins. Each housewife had towels which were dampened and used to swab off sticky faces and fingers after the meal was over. And of course no one would think of coming to a Fourth of July celebration without a clean handkerchief.

The meal was a merry one, but there was no dawdling over food, and in less than an hour from the time the first preparations were made, Mrs. Evans was wheedling someone please to take just one piece from her last pie—to have a pie left uncut was a sure sign that people didn't like her pies. Which argument was speedily put to rout by jolly references to the two that had disappeared almost without a trace.

While the women cleared away the dishes and the remains of the food, the men lounged about on the grass and smoked—pipes and cigars only. No respectable man of affairs smoked cigarettes. Cigarette smoking was supposed to be limited to shifty-eyed underworld personalities. "Coffin nails" we called them, and whenever I saw a youth with a cigarette I could imagine him with his hands palsied, his face thin and sallow; I could see him literally shriveling away into the grave. (A prime example of an idea which detoured widely, then returned finally to its original concept.)

The children disappeared again immediately after dinner.

"Now don't spend all your money on the shooting gallery and the merry-go-round, and don't make yourselves sick eating too much stuff," Mother admonished the boys as they left.

"What shall we spend our money for, then?" Floyd asked, leaving her helpless for a reply. The Fourth was just one day in the year, after all, and they were pretty good boys, I could sense her arguing with herself. Maybe she needn't worry too much about what they did.

The twins liked to go about with me, and I promised to look after them for the afternoon. This was not altogether big-sister benevolence on my part. I was really glad to do so. I felt I was too old to be interested in some of their juvenile pleasures, and having some little girls with me gave me an excuse to enjoy them vicariously. So, as long as our money lasted, we walked up and down, saw all the sights, played games, bought a toy monkey on a stick, popcorn, sea foam candy and ice cream, and rode on the merry-go-round. The twins' vitality was exhausted at about the same time, although they would not admit it, and when mother met us again she took them with her to sit in the park.

None of the children ate much supper. They would have preferred to skip the meal altogether, to continue their feasting on knickknacks and excitement, but were restrained by firm parental dicta, the summary of which were, "You've got to settle down for awhile anyway, or you'll be so plumb wore out you won't be able to stay awake to watch the fireworks." The more habit addicted adults adhered to the routine of supper, a snack affair of leftovers eaten with the fingers, including the rest of Mrs. Evan's pie.

After supper there was an interval of impatient waiting until dark, when we would go back to the park to watch the fireworks. There was really no good reason for going to the park, father contended; with no trees and no tall buildings to obscure vision, we couldn't help seeing them wherever we were. But the park was where the crowds would be, and there were benches to sit on, so the park was where all the rest of us wanted to go. After an hour of the soaring excitement of brave pyrotechnics we went back to the tents to bed. The children all preferred to sleep out in the open, so their beds were easily improvised of horse blankets spread on the grass. Men and women were segregated in the two tents, on similar beds, arranged by the light of a lantern in each tent.

"I don't know whether I can stand another two days of

this or not," Mrs. Evans said after we were all settled and she blew out the lantern in our tent. I held my breath as mother agreed with her, thankful that father was not within hearing distance of such discussion. I prayed that such a thought would not occur to him, for a decision by father that one day of this orgy was enough would be final, fatal. The next morning, however, everybody seemed rested and in good spirits, and there was not a word spoken of surfeit.

The big feature at the park that morning was the wedding of a local couple in the bandstand, and an imposing display of wedding gifts given by Dallas merchants to promote the public ceremony. "What else will they think of?" people asked. The answers were prolonged throughout that day and the next, a continuing round of athletic contests, races, feats of bronco-busting, tent shows, band concerts, and parades.

By the end of the second day we children had spent all our money, and Father gave us an extra quarter apiece after breakfast the next morning, with the admonition that we should be back in the schoolhouse yard ready to start home by three o'clock. I spent my quarter for something I had been coveting for the entire three days, a fan of transparent silk with Japanese ladies painted on it in colors, stretched tightly over a frame with a black lacquered handle with a silk tassel.

"I can't think of anything I would have spent my whole quarter for," Fern said, disapprovingly. He still had a dime left.

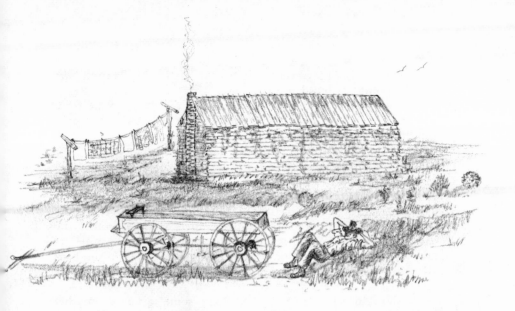

7 | THE SOD HOUSE FAMILY

ON THE DAY AFTER our extended Fourth of July holiday, the boys were getting ready to go fishing after dinner.

"Fishing doesn't seem as exciting as it used to," Fern remarked, and Floyd agreed with him. None of the rest of us was going with them. Mother was baking bread, the twins wanted to play with their dolls after their three-day absence, and I planned to wash my hair.

Floyd glanced up from the fishing line he was trying to untangle, and exclaimed excitedly, "Look! There's two rigs coming down from the Smith hill!"

Two vehicles on the road past our house at the same time were an almost unheard of amount of traffic. We all stopped what we were doing and watched them approach. Father even delayed getting back to his plowing to watch with us.

"Probably some Nebraska farmers coming back from hauling grain to Gregory," mother said.

"There's not likely any grain being sold this time of year," father reminded her.

The vehicles were lumber wagons, each pulled by a team of mules, and they were followed by four lanky hounds. Before they were quite opposite our house, they turned off to the right, stopped, and began unloading a tent and other gear indistinguishable to us. These gestures of occupancy identified them immediately.

"They're our new neighbors!" father exclaimed. "It's the

Missouri family they were telling me about in Paxton, and they're going to build a sod house."

Their arrival made quite a cavalcade. There were the three wagons containing machinery, tools, and household goods; a small herd of cattle; several saddle ponies; and too many hounds to count accurately since they kept darting about under the wagons and among the cattle. These hounds were so thin mother said they looked like rabbits that had been skinned.

Father, accompanied by the boys, went across the road to talk to them before going to the field, and reported some brief details to us. They were the Langenfelders from Missouri, and they were, indeed, building a sod house. The boys wanted to stay and play with the hounds, but father made them come back with him, to insure that they would not be a nuisance to the new arrivals.

"Shouldn't I offer to cook them some dinner?" mother asked. "It's only a little after one, and they surely haven't eaten." But father said he had already asked them, and they had refused. They had some lunch with them, and were just getting ready to eat it.

The boys gave up all idea of fishing for the afternoon, too interested in what the new neighbors were doing. We had seen a number of sod houses, but none of us had ever seen one being built. The boys were disappointed they didn't get right at it that very afternoon, but the men seemed in no hurry. They spent the afternoon unloading the wagons, setting up a tent, and moving things inside it. Then they smoked their pipes for awhile, and finally lay down on the grass and took a nap in the shade of the tent.

The building of the soddy started the next day, and the boys, the twins, and I were daily spectators of this piece of construction. There was hardly a piece of sod laid in those walls that some of us did not see.

A sod house is made by piling pieces of sod one upon another in much the same manner as bricks are laid except that no sealing substance such as mortar is needed. The sod is turned over by the breaking plow in flat pieces about a foot wide, in varying lengths depending upon where the strip breaks as it is turned over. The walls are built up snugly from the earth, leaving no opportunity for the wind to blow under the floor, thus making a sod house a much warmer one than the average claim shack built of lumber, with no foundation. (Claim shacks like ours had to be "banked" for the winter, usually with the horse manure mixed with straw that was cleaned daily from the floor of the barn. This was not so disagreeable as it sounds, resulting in a frozen, impermeable, protective mass, odorless so long as it remained frozen.)

The men worked steadily every day, there being little rain at this season to interrupt their labors. They moved slowly and deliberately—"moseying," father called it, while the four hounds lay under the wagons and watched them, with occasional sniffing, barking forays into the surrounding prairie, on the trail of ground squirrels, jack rabbits, or prairie dogs. Father said he didn't see how they would ever have a roof over their heads before winter at the rate they were going. But they did finish by late summer and went to bring their families who had halted somewhere with friends on their way up from Missouri. Completed, the house was an elongated building of one room, with a board floor laid inside, and a board roof. Turning a solid back against the blizzardy north, its southern exposure had one door, and four windows opened on the east, west, and south.

It was not claim country etiquette to wait until a new family was settled and curtains hung at the windows, before making the first neighborly call. The possibility that helpful services could be rendered to a new family a long way from home took precedence over other considerations. So when mother saw several little children running about she went right over. Having five children of her own, she knew that in moving time it can be quite a help to have the little ones looked after apart from the scene of operations. She brought only two little girls back with her, however. The younger children were very shy, and threatened to raise quite a hullabaloo if she insisted upon bringing them.

The advent of these two little girls, Maudie and Ida, seven and eight years old, was the beginning of our acquaintance with the Langenfelder family, so different from any of the other Dakota settlers. The heads of the family were a triumvirate of brothers: Zeke, Luke, and Barth. Zeke, the oldest, was a bachelor; the other two had wives and families. Their complete family circle, with no visiting relatives present, numbered twelve persons. Mother would not believe, at first, that the entire group planned to live there in that one-room house. She thought that surely only one family would be living there, that the others had accompanied them to help get them settled and the barn built, before winter. We were assured, however, that it was to be home for all of them.

Accommodating themselves to their cramped quarters was a matter of getting along with what they had. The stove, table, chairs, and cupboard occupied the central portion of the house, into which the one door opened. The ends were curtained off into bedrooms. During the daytime these curtains were pushed back, and the beds served as lounging places for men, dogs, and children. The women never did much lounging. The dogs numbered seven or eight, all told, and they all had fleas. The adults in the family thought little of this circumstance; they were accustomed to the fleas and had acquired some adeptness in fighting them off. Among the younger members, being bitten by fleas was one of the usual afflictions of childhood.

Winnie, wife of Luke, the second brother, was the member of the family whom I came to know best. She had an irresponsible, uncomplaining temperament, and accepted her lot in life with unbelievable acquiescence. Always there was enough work to do in a day to keep her occupied, and troubles that might come tomorrow were nothing that she worried about today. Not that a life of labor was any less the lot of the other pioneer women, but they were supplied with tools of some degree of adequacy with which to do it and she was not. The others had hopes and dreams for the future which sustained them. Whatever dreams poor Winnie may have had must have been in the nature of fantasies for surely she could have had no real hope for anything other than a continued poverty-stricken existence.

Winnie's older daughter, Maudie, looked a great deal like her, and there seemed to be a rapport between them. This child had the habit of going off into hysterical fits of giggling at times, for no apparent reason. This was extremely disconcerting to anyone within her hearing, except her mother, in whose mind this moronic gaiety seemed to pass for brief spasms of happiness.

Maudie, Ida, and their little brother Joe were shy, staring, backward creatures, with a fascinatingly ungrammatical speech which the twins were soon imitating until father reprimanded them sternly for it several times. They never looked grossly dirty, but always untidy, perhaps because they wore such an odd assortment of clothes. When we first became acquainted with them they were wearing stiff, high, button shoes, the like of which I had seen even in pictures only once in my life, and that was in some old copies of *Chatterbox*. These shoes were quite new, and the little girls were proud of them, Ida confiding in us that a nice "store man" had given the shoes to them. That marked the people, in my eyes, as being of another class. We had never dreamed, then, of anything like our present-day relief programs, and the people who had clothes given to them promiscuously were shiftless and incapable of managing well.

Aside from the sporadic and haphazard farming operations carried on by the brothers, it was upon Winnie's shoulders that the manual labor of the household fell. She did practically all the washing, ironing, and scrubbing. She milked the cows when "the boys" felt too tired, or if milk was needed before they were up in the morning. She chopped kindling when there was any to chop, and made long forays into the surrounding prairie to pick up for fuel the flat cow chips of dried dung from the range cattle. The Langenfelder women felt it to be their duty to keep their menfolk and children clothed, warm, and fed, whether any adequate wherewithal was provided or not. If they ever reproached their indolent men for lack of proper support, we never heard of it. Once when they had insufficient fuel to finish cooking dinner, we saw Winnie go out and saw off the surplus from the tops of a number of fence posts, for wood to burn.

When they were out of food they would often borrow. Their intentions about paying it back were genuinely good, I am sure, but the occasions when they had a sufficient surplus to allow for the returning of any to a neighbor were quite rare. It was a not uncommon occurrence for them to send a child to borrow a loaf of bread for dinner, and then send another child to borrow another loaf before the meal was over. Mother soon found it advisable to be conveniently out of whatever they came to borrow but she was unable to follow this rule very consistently. She couldn't bear to think of the children going hungry. She knew, too, that either of the Langenfelder women would have shared a last crust with her.

Winnie had one peculiar sensitive point, difficult to understand. She regarded her feet as too hideously large, was very much ashamed of them, and tried to wear shoes of as small size as possible. She was a large-boned woman, with good musculature and a good figure, in general, and I do not recall that her feet were larger than a woman of her build might expect to have. But she thought them so, and the thought was a real pain to her. Her hands were large and conspicuously red and rough from labor, but apparently they never worried her. In fact, mother was horrified once to go to the Langenfelder house and find Winnie scrubbing the floor, stepping about on two blocks of wood to do so. She explained that she was using pretty strong lye water, and didn't want it to eat the soles of her shoes. Yet she was putting her hands into it! Her obsession about her feet probably had its origin in descriptions of fragile, fainting heroines in novels she had read, in whose footsteps the poor woman may have followed in her daydreams. It was true that the shoes she wore never made her feet look any better, for much of the time she did not own a presentable pair, and she often went about wearing some of the men's old work shoes.

Winnie's sister-in-law, Evie, wife of Barth, the youngest

brother, was a frail little woman, with braids of graying dark hair wound around her head. She must have been pretty once. She gave the impression of having memories of past attractions, which gave her a certain air, although few of these youthful attractions remained. Her face was gaunt, her skin becoming wrinkled ,and saggy, and her winsome smile showed teeth that were becoming carious. Her husband, Barth, was still handsome, in an indolent sort of way. Evie had had an illegitimate child before her marriage, a girl who lived with Evie's parents, and came to visit her mother occasionally. Her presence seemed to irritate Barth, and she was not the type to mollify such irritation, being a loud, brazen little vixen who appeared to have burst from childhood into womanhood, fullblown. One wondered whether Evie's slavish devotion to Barth was not born of gratitude for his having taken her, a fallen woman, so graciously under his roof.

Evie was the manager of the household. It was she who eked out what they had to cover their needs as nearly as possible; her task to plan so that each child had clothes to cover him. The bulk of the heavy work fell upon Winnie, not because Evie was indolent, or a shirker, but because Winnie was physically able to endure more of the grilling, slavish, indecently driving labor that visibly wore them both out. Yet they always seemed happy and cheerful, and it would be difficult to imagine two sisters-in-law living in the same house and maintaining a more harmonious relationship with each other.

Neither of these women appeared to see any fault in their menfolk. They could look up from their steaming washtubs with all the pride in the world, and watch the men ride grandly away on a coyote or jack rabbit hunt, followed by the pack of yelping hounds. If they brought home several jack rabbits for tomorrow's dinner, that was their full duty.

When the children needed clothes, and there was no money for materials, as there frequently was not, they dyed flour sacks to make dresses for the girls and shirts for the boys. The particular shades of red and blue dye that they used came to be associated rather unpleasantly in my mind with the Langenfelder children, like the uniforms of an institution. Evie's children always had "something decent to put on," some garment apiece that was whole, and halfway presentable. Winnie's children often did not. Evie had a little more general pride; such things were a little more important to her. When the new school house was built, and Sunday school was started in it, Evie sent her older children, but Winnie's children could not go; they literally had nothing to wear.

Evie had a number of children after they moved to the claim. She seemed always to be nursing one infant, or expecting another. It was heartbreaking to see her wispy, aging little body undergoing such a constant drain. She never had a doctor when any of these children were born. They called mother to come and take care of her. Mother had never done such a thing before, but there was no refusing such necessity. Other neighbors were farther away, and Winnie would have panicked at the thought of undertaking a task of such delicacy and importance. So mother, tutored only by her own personal experiences in childbirth and what father could tell her about deliveries of young farm animals, acted as midwife. No child ever arrived in Evie's rapidly swelling family without some pitiful show of welcome. Mother once said that it made her feel like crying to see poor, tired Evie embroidering french knots in a little flour-sack dress for a new baby that was coming.

The Langenfelders had one unbelievably incongruous possession, a herd of purebred Jersey cattle. How such a family came to accumulate a herd of blooded stock, no one could imagine. Finding some sterling silver or a piece of Royal Doulton china in their house could not have been much more startling. In father's opinion the Jersey breed of cattle was all wrong for that country, but however that may have been, the Langenfelder family were all extremely proud of them, probably the only possession they had ever had which others might regard with envy. They loved to speak of the cows by name, and gloried in the ferocity of Old Ike, the bull. Old Ike was a terror to us all. We never ventured far without making sure he was not on the loose. His disposition was sometimes transmitted to his offspring. We owned a calf sired by him that was vicious from babyhood. He would attack with gusto anyone who came near. Mother was afraid even to feed him. He ended in veal at a precocious age.

Another incongruous feature of the Langenfelder family was that they all read voraciously, especially the men, since the women had so much less time. But thirst for knowledge, love of literature, desire for self-improvement—none of these motives was involved. Their reading was on a par with their aimless whittling, mumbletypeg, spitting tobacco juice—amusing ways of killing time. They had piles of battered, half-worn-out copies of *Diamond Dick, Lady Southworth, Mary J. Holmes,* and others of the ilk that mother and father were wont to put together, scathingly, into one execrable class, "dime novels." I borrowed many of these books, which I was able to read by virtue of the fact that mother was too busy with a multitude of other things always to know the name of the book I was reading. When she did happen to notice any of these lurid titles, however, the book ended then and there, as far as I was concerned. This happened in the case of *Darkness and Daylight,* which I was required to return immediately. I was forbidden ever to finish it, and for weeks I thought I should never be happy without knowing how that book ended.

Full to capacity as the Langenfelder house appeared to be, it was to have additional tenants for the winter. This was to be Granny's home, too, Evie told us. Granny had always lived with them, had been spending the summer with another son until the house was ready. Granny was the matriarch of the household, mother of the Langenfelder men of whom she was very proud. To her, there was nothing disgraceful about their lying about the house in the daytime—reading, smoking, playing with the hounds. She beamed upon them benignly, believing them as nearly perfect as mortals get to be.

Granny smoked a cob pipe as regularly as her sons did, but not so openly. Getting out of her Missouri hills, she learned that most women did not smoke—not even cigarettes, at that time—and that a woman smoking a pipe was a curiosity. So she always thrust her pipe out of sight somewhere when a stranger came in. Well acquainted with us as she became, she never smoked in our presence, but would hide her pipe under her apron or in the chair behind her until we were gone, causing the other occupants of the room much general uneasiness about the possibility of fire. She was a skinny, leathery little woman, no longer very active. She would sit close to the fire, smoking or dozing, or sometimes minding the latest baby for brief intervals, preferring to keep out of the way of the bustling younger women. The bustling part of her life was over, and this was her reward, to sit in the place of honor and keep a tolerant eye on the teeming lives of the generations that followed her.

Two other regular winter residents in the Langenfelder home were the Bunton boys, Dixon and Lang, cousins of the Langenfelder brothers. They had no people of their own, these being their nearest relatives. Winnie and Evie were very proud of these cousins by marriage, and always accorded them a warm welcome. They were handsome men and carried themselves with an indolent variety of dash. They brought presents for everyone and made contributions of small luxuries from time to time throughout the winter.

Lang, the elder Bunton, was a smooth, secretive, reserved man. His attitude toward other men was gracious but wary and there was a speculative gleam in his eyes when he looked at women. Quiet as he was, he still gave the impression of being always on the alert. No one seemed to have a very good idea of how Lang occupied himself when he was not in winter quarters. No one spoke of the work he was engaged in, but whatever he did was sufficiently remunerative to permit him to dress very well and to supply himself with a generous amount of spending money throughout the winter. He was always armed, but we never knew him to fire his gun, even at targets. While he was lounging about, however, his hand would make a graceful sweep to his holster from time to time, as if he were routinely keeping a certain motion in practice. Ingenuously, I once asked Winnie pointblank what kind of job Lang had. She replied uneasily that she did not know; that he often mentioned having business in various places but never said just what it was. She thought the boys knew something about his work, but never liked to have the women ask questions about it.

Dixon Bunton was a handsome, statuesque, bronzed youth of twenty. He was a cowboy, and I think without exception the most romantic figure I ever knew in the flesh, romance being so much more a quality of the mind envisioning it than of the corporeal subject of the visions. He was the idol of the young femininity of the entire countryside, on a par with the screen figures who came later to entrance the minds of young girls and of many women old enough to know better. It was an important social event when Dixon Bunton came back for the winter. He rode a fine, spirited saddle horse, and with his jingling spurs, his silk shirt and neckerchief, his soft, broad-rimmed hat, and his easy grace in the saddle, was a figure to be gazed after by almost any female. He was supposed at that time to be enamoured of a young Indian girl who lived near his range; but that did not prevent his casting a roving eye about, to see what this country offered. He carried a gun, too; was a fine shot, and loved to display his marksmanship.

A social event graced by the presence of Dixon Bunton was an affair no girl cared to miss. Once at a box social at the schoolhouse, Winnie had assured me that he intended to buy my box. I think I had never really believed that such a dazzling piece of fortune would come to me, and it was well that I had not. For I suffered the agony of seeing this god fall to the lot of one of the Randall girls, while a married man, thirty-five if he was a day, bought my box. Winnie explained afterward that it had been unavoidable on Dixon's part; that he had been sitting beside the Randall girl's brother who had urged him to buy his sister's box, and he could hardly refuse to do so without appearing rude. However that may have been, it was a heartbreaking incident at the time. Yet, curiously enough, there was a measure of relief in it, too. I was painfully shy, and having to eat supper with such a personage would probably have made me tongue-tied, unable to talk or eat with any ease. I should have been quite as comfortable sitting beside King Arthur.

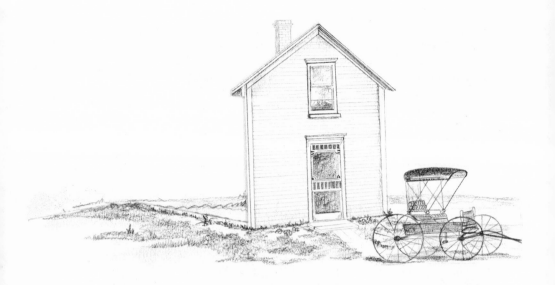

8 / OUR ENGLISH FRIENDS

THE SMITH FAMILY, who lived a mile and a half north of us, were as extraordinary as the Langenfelders in many exactly opposite respects. They were intelligent, industrious, provident, honest, and farseeing. These were, indeed, qualities shared by most of the other homesteaders, but the Smiths remained different from all the rest in spite of these points of similarity. I was about to say that they had not been long enough out of England to lose the patina of the mother country. But for how many generations must an Englishman be expatriate for this to happen? This is a question difficult to answer, for I doubt it ever happens in its entirety. I have always had a high regard for England, and felt much warmth toward its people. Until the time of this writing, I had never asked myself when or how this feeling began, but it may very well have had its origin in my acquaintanceship with the Smith family. If it had been present before, knowing them surely strengthened it. I have never lost this affection for the English. When I grew up I married one, which added greatly to my knowledge of their quirks and oddities but left the basic structure of my regard unchanged.

Our acquaintance with the Smiths began while they were still living in their barn, during the time the house was being built. They had made themselves quite cozy and comfortable in their temporary quarters, and received visitors there with as much grace and geniality as any hosts ever did in an orthodox dwelling. Four children were in the family, but the older two, Bert and Helen, were away much of the time, being employed at their previous residence in Nebraska. We came to know the younger two, Harold and Edith, very well, and Floyd and I became close friends with them.

Their house was finished late in the summer and was a larger one than most of the other settlers had. It was built not with any idea of being pretentious but because they thought they needed it—it was as necessary to have space for a piano and books as for the requisite number of chairs and beds.

Mr. Smith was a frail, dreamy, impractical man, about as poorly adapted to the rigors of pioneer life as one could imagine. While he read, dreamed, and philosophized, his wife and children carried on the homesteading venture. They made an excellent job of it, considering the fact that they had never lived on a farm before. They read books about farming, were sharply alert in their observations, and asked questions of their neighbors. Out of all this they developed their own methods of procedure on what seemed to them the most sensible plan. Whether it was orthodox never bothered them.

The father had his place in their scheme of things, too, although his contribution to the family accomplishments was of a more ethereal nature. They looked to him a great deal for inspiration and encouragement and to provide the tone for the family ideals. His frail person could hardly have contributed anything of a strenuous physical nature. He read copiously, daily, and while his wife and children were busy battling for a living in this untried land, he would be engrossed happily in *The Boer War,* or other favorites. He and I were once contestants in a spelling bee at the sod schoolhouse. We were the only ones left standing, when I went down to defeat by putting an *e* instead of an *i* in the middle of "privilege," leaving him the victor.

It goes without saying that Mr. Smith was something of an enigma to the other homesteaders. They found him difficult to talk to or to understand. He became, therefore, a figure of amusement to them (though perhaps not so unwittingly as they believed). Relating the latest odd thing that gentle Mr. Smith had said or done often added merriment to gatherings of the more roughneck Dakotans. One of these stories concerned the mules, Dolly and Dora, the chief work team of the Smiths. Mr. Smith was helping some of the neighbors haul rocks to fill a gully in the road. Within a few yards of their destination Dora balked. With legs braced and ears laid back, she refused to move another step. The other men left their wagons standing and gathered about to watch developments. How would this mild-mannered Englishman deal with such a situation? Did he know enough cuss words to get him out of it (swearing being the traditionally accepted way of dealing with a balky mule)? Mr. Smith descended slowly from his wagon and walked around to the front of his team. Then he shook his head and said sadly, "Oh Dora, Dora! You do vex me so!"

To my brothers and me, the Smith home was an oasis in a vast bookless desert. Walking up to their house to return books we had borrowed, and to get others, became a regular pilgrimage for us. Dickens, Chaucer, Thackeray, Macaulay, Shakespeare, Spenser—they had all these and derived a second pleasure from them in seeing them thus enjoyed by others. I am everlastingly indebted to them for their generosity, and, as with so many favors given in this world, my gratitude is much more deeply appreciative now in my mature years than it was at the time. One winter I read the complete works of Dickens, borrowing them all from the Smiths. My earliest knowledge of the old Egyptian dynasties came from some book I borrowed there, the name of which I have forgotten. It was in a book of theirs, too, that I first met "Black Douglas." I sat up one night after everyone else had gone to bed to finish reading *Dr. Jekyll and Mr. Hyde*, and by the time I had completed it I was so saturated with horror that I was afraid to blow out the lamp and go to bed, so I curled up in my chair beside the stove, leaned my head on the table, and slept until morning. But all these are merely isolated little islands in the vast sea of reading with which this family supplied me.

Novices as they were at pioneering, in another sense the Smiths were recognized leaders in the community. No neighborhood plan, organization, or entertainment was complete without the Smiths in it. They were talented, versatile, and cooperative. There was little money or opportunity for music lessons among the pioneers, but from lessons learned in her own youth Mrs. Smith taught her older daughter, and Helen in turn taught Edith. With the finishing lessons she obtained later when she went away to school, Edith became an accomplished musician. The entire Smith family sang at home in the evenings, and could always be depended upon, with very short notice, to have a well-practiced duet, trio, or quartet number. A solo from Harold was almost taken for granted when any program was being prepared. He usually sang lyrics or ballads, but one night he brought the house down more riotously than usual with his rendition of "Who Put the Overalls in Mrs. Murphy's Chowder?" When a new organ was purchased for the schoolhouse,

Edith automatically became the organist for church and Sunday school. When a play was planned for the literary society, Mrs. Smith was called upon to coach it. If a script had been lacking, she probably could have written one.

Their home, too, became a recognized center for social activities. They were simply and wholeheartedly hospitable, and we loved to spend an afternoon or evening with them. They were all interesting conversationalists, and had a large fund of subjects for discourse, never needing to rely upon gossip or other small-minded trivia. Relatives in England and in Canada were always sending them books, magazines, snapshots, and bundles of newspapers. There would be chatty letters, too, from these same people, excerpts from which might be read to us, giving us little glimpses into other worlds. It occurs to me now, although it did not then, that the letters the Smiths wrote to these relatives in return must have seemed to them as wildly unreal as messages from the moon.

Being invited to supper at the Smiths' house was always a treat; sometimes we had food we had never tasted before, such as roast guinea fowl, or some of Mrs. Smith's own make of marmalade, but it was not only the food that was different. A meal there was something more than food. It was a festive occasion, garnished with good food; a leisurely time of stimulating conversation, with exercises in wit and repartee. "Dawdling" thus at the table was unheard of in our own home, and we found it enjoyable, as straitlaced people often enjoy practices they regard as racy or faintly sinful.

Trying to convey completely the sphere of influence of such a family as this, is difficult indeed, but my life was certainly influenced by their civility and grace.

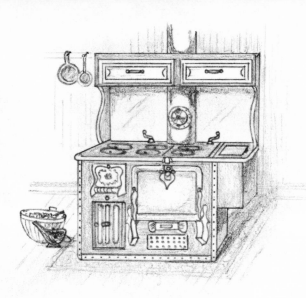

9 / GRACES AND DIVERSIONS

ON THE TOP SHELF of a china cabinet in my house stands a large Haviland china platter, a beautiful piece, with a gold band around the edge, and decorated with misty sprays of pink flowers. It is one of the few survivors of the hundred piece set that went with us to the claim in South Dakota, probably one of the most incongruous furnishings in any of these pioneer houses. It was as out of place in this rugged environment as the Langenfelders' herd of Jersey cattle. Father had urged strongly that this china be sold, but the thought was so heartbreaking to mother that he relented and helped her pack it. This set of dishes had a sentimental value to her, in addition to the fondness most women have for beautiful china. It had been bought with part of a small legacy from her mother.

Impractical as they were, I think father did well to compromise on taking the dishes. Mother had given up enough, as it was, of those things so much more important to a woman than to a man; such things as rugs and upholstered chairs that were outside the realm of stark utility and faintly tinged with luxury. The parlor organ was probably the most difficult of anything for mother to leave behind. She had had it the longest of any of her possessions, having bought it from Montgomery Ward before she was married with the proceeds from the sale of a pig her father had given her to raise. She sold the organ to Mrs. McBride for five dollars, an initial investment in the musical education of Mrs. McBride's son, Hobart.

This organ was more than a musical instrument; it was the ornamental piece in the "front room." It had little mirrors,

70

patches of red plush set behind grillworks of polished wood, platforms with fences around them to make protected shelves for bric-a-brac, carvings and curvettings, turrets and cupolas, all of which ended in a sweep of grandeur almost at the ceiling.

Mother played by ear, and the pleasantest memory associated with that old organ is of her playing and singing to us in the evening before the lamp was lit, while we were waiting for father to come home to supper. She sang hymns mostly, and ballads. There was one about Pontchartrain, a lover's account of his sweetheart's freezing to death—"and my mind went back to the time she said, 'I'm growing warmer now,'" a grim reference to the fact that a freezing person loses the sense of pain at the onset of death. It gave me quite a thrill in later years to learn that there really is a Lake Pontchartrain, like something come to reality that I had long believed a myth (although if the ballad referred to the lake in Louisiana, it does seem a most unlikely setting for someone freezing to death). There was one ballad that told of a settler's coming home to find that all his family had been massacred by the Indians; in this ballad, someone had "turned and closed the garden gate" before going out to meet his fate.

There was nothing in this latter ballad that seemed unlikely to any of us. It probably contributed to mother's trepidation about the Indians of Dakota, although her own previous association with Indians had been with peaceful, friendly ones. The most fascinating stories mother ever told us, better than any fairy tales, were the series, "when we came west from Clinton County." How they rode in covered wagons, the boys on horseback, driving the cattle; how they did their cooking over camp fires, and what they ate; building the log house; the terrific blizzards during which, snug beside a roaring fire, they sewed carpet rags and knitted their own stockings. Interspersed in all this were accounts of meeting with Indians, from none of whom they ever met any hostility. One thing she told us about them was that they never invited any whites to eat with them. If white visitors lingered until mealtime, they were told politely to "puckachee," which meant "go home." The only time I ever saw this word in print was in MacKinlay Kantor's book, *Arouse and Beware.* I had always understood it to be "puckagee" but I am sure the Kantor version is the correct one, knowing how painstakingly he does research for his books.

Their log house was built within walking distance of the railroad, and one of the diversions of mother and her sisters was to go down to the railroad and watch for a certain passenger train to go by. In this way they made the visual acquaintance of the porter on the dining car, who would watch for them and wave to them with a broad smile, thus extending their racial knowledge to include negroes as well as Indians, finding both colors equally friendly and kind. One day the porter threw a little package out to them as the train passed. In it were several limes, the first they had ever seen, and a packet of sugar, with a note saying, "For the little girls to make lemonade of."

Mother's china was more than a set of dishes to her, more than usefulness, or even beauty. They were a tangible link, a reminder, that there are refinements of living difficult to perpetuate in rugged frontier conditions, perhaps in danger of being forgotten. Even with the dishes to remind and encourage her, it was difficult for mother to adhere to practices she thought proper when father was away. Father's absences were apt to be considered by all of us children, especially the boys, as a time for lapse from formalities or even an occasion for some rowdyism. Whenever father was away for a meal, mother would insist that Floyd say grace. Whatever reverence Floyd had in him was apt to come out with a rollicking overlay. Once we had for supper in father's absence, some navy beans boiled with a hambone, and no other prepared food. Floyd looked at the one hot dish on the table, and as we all bowed our heads he said, in a voice vibrant with fervor, "Dear Lord, are we ever thankful for these beans!"

Individual resources of strength and contentment were never dredged more nearly to the depths than on the long winter evenings when we were isolated in our too closely packed little house, with no possible means of communication with the outside world except by travel, which on the stormy nights was not to be thought of. The only forays we made outside the house on such nights were the necessary ones, to take care of the stock, bring in water and fuel, and to "go out," which was our stark euphemism for a visit to the privy, some little distance from the house, with not even a path shoveled to it, most likely, as the path would have been drifted full of snow again before the shoveler had finished his task.

As far as possible, evening chores would have been done before dark; thus avoiding the added burden of carrying a lantern. Coal and kindling for the morning fire would have been brought in, and a pailful of water, perhaps two, from the well. The water would be a cylinder of ice by morning, with the dipper imprisoned in it. By the time the last of the chores were done, and father came back into the house and took off his heavy wraps, the moisture in his breath would be frozen into little icicles on the ends of his moustache.

Foods vulnerable to cold, such as potatoes and other vegetables and canned fruit, must remain in the cave overnight, not the kitchen, or they would be ruined. Sometimes even the bread would be frozen and the hard slices would have an icy sheen to them when cut. These remained very palatable, however, when thawed in the oven or in a steamer on top of the stove. We had not yet learned about toast. One of the earliest comments I ever heard about toast was that of a neighbor whose daughter had gone to work for a family outside the state. "They eat burned bread for breakfast," she reported.

After the first year, when we had built a small addition to the house, we added a luxury that was beyond comparison to anything we had yet known, a base burner. This was a stove that burned hard coal, broken into pebble-sized pieces which could be put into the stove in hoppersful and fed automatically into the fire, much like the stokers used in basement furnaces later. A fire burning in the house all night! It was wonderful! Not a roaring fire, it is true, but definitely a warm spot; and warmer still, the psychological effect of seeing the glow through the isinglass windows of the firebox.

Coming home late—maybe even as late as eleven—on a cold night, the thought of the waiting fire was, in itself, a warming one. We were likely to be walking home. The schoolhouse, built in our second year, a half-mile north of us, was the common gathering spot for neighborhood affairs—church, box socials, spelling bees, holiday festivities. Father always said it was better for us to walk that short distance than to have the horses standing out in the cold, a chilling session for them, even protected with their horseblankets and tied on the side of the schoolhouse most sheltered from the wind.

So we would walk, bundled in our heaviest, warmest clothes, so necessary and at the same time so awkward in their weight, stumbling along in the deep snow, no part of the road cleared, so that keeping to the right route was guesswork, turning at times and trying to walk backward to give our faces a respite from the freezing wind, but making such slow progress because of frequent falling that we soon turned back again, shielding our faces with our mittened hands. On a clear night, with moonlight, our house was easily visible from the schoolhouse, but on a stormy night, with the air full of blowing snow, we had to be almost upon it to see even the faint glow from the front windows. The glow meant a welcoming warmth once we were inside the door; its meaning was heat, not light. No one ever left a kerosene lamp burning in an empty house, for fear of fire. Once inside, we were back again in the warm shelter of home, to a contentment that was never expressed in words, only felt.

The most nearly regular neighborhood meeting held at

the schoolhouse was what we called a "literary," not a literary anything, just a "literary," using the adjective as a noun in this instance, as I have heard the verb "sing" used as a noun in the sense of a community song festival. Weather permitting, we had a literary every Friday night during the winter. There was a program committee for each week, with whom absolute cooperation was the rule. Everyone in the neighborhood was expected to contribute his bit of talent, in turn, when called upon. No one was privileged to sit back and listen for a winter without taking his turn at performing. To do so would be to lose face. For many it was a painful ordeal, but to go through with it was preferable to staying away from the meetings. Miss a whole winter's entertainment? It was not to be thought of. The productions forthcoming were varied, original, and sometimes quite startling, and no star on the professional stage was ever applauded more heartily than one of these performers when he had risen nobly to do his duty.

There were vehement debates on political, moral, philosophical, but usually nonsensical subjects—resolved that the cow is more useful to man than the horse (the horse having much more going for him then, when he was our chief source of power); that pigs are smarter than sheep; that it is better to be kicked by a mule than bitten by a rattler. There was always a liberal sprinkling of "speaking pieces." Into this group fell many with no special talents, as anyone was supposed to be able to "speak a piece." Henri Mignery, our dark little Frenchman, rather shy, brought down the house one night with his rendition of "I had a brother, and his name was Ike. Came all the way from Missouri, all the way from the Pike," and so on, for a liberal dozen verses full of harrowing experiences. Father's contribution was a series of narrative rhymes, composed to order, about local people and incidents. One of these came to be an expected number on every program.

Occasionally there was a play, a rare and special treat. Plays were difficult to manage; it was too arduous and uncertain an undertaking to plan for the players to get together over bad roads, for rehearsals. Mrs. Smith attempted a pageant once, with the title "The Queen of Roses." This, however, was too nicely sentimental for the taste of the young bloods who were to take part in it, and when, at the dress rehearsal, they put pepper in the paper roses they waved over the sleeping queen, she gave up the project in disgust.

For each literary evening there was one journalism number. One person was assigned the preparation of a newspaper composed mostly of personal items about the people present. Many of these items were pure fabrications; others contained more truth than delicacy. Nothing was sacred from the pens of these editors, who usually had old scores to pay from previous productions of other editors. Love affairs were the choicest material. Any joke on an individual was literally worn out in these pages. Fantastic and horrifying horoscopes were read, and romantic and opulent futures foretold for the Rosebud Country.

Music was always a greatly appreciated form of entertainment, for musical talent was not plentiful. A fiddle or accordion number was a prize, and lustily applauded as long as more was forthcoming. I have attempted to describe what a shining light the Smith family was in our community. Here they shone literally, in public, their talents pinpointed for our delectation. Edith was always the accompanist for any musical number, and songs were always expected from some or all of the rest of the family. Mr. Smith's preference was for old English ballads. A favorite of Harold's contained the lines, "And there's ne'er a gossoon in the village, Dares tread on the tail of me coat." Songs such as "My Little Old Sod Shanty on the Claim," and "For I'm a Young Cowboy, And I Know I've Done Wrong" (although I do not recall the sin that was the source of his lament) were enjoyed over and over. They never wore out.

One night the Runkel and the Shepard girls sang "Casey Jones," and they were applauded with such fervor that they had to repeat it several times. I have no idea how old the song was at that time, but it was the first time any of us had heard it. A piece of new sheet music was a treasure. Such a possession classed one as up-to-date, one of the smart set. Popular songs were a long time reaching us, and some of them never did. No professional entertainers ever came to us; even news of them and their offerings was a rarity. Letters, newspapers, and magazines were our only means of communication with the outside world, and they were not plentiful. One of the things that intrigued me on a trip to Alaska in recent years was that Alaskans were wont to refer to anything outside their state, or territory, as it was then, as being "on the outside." A trip to the main body of the United States was a trip "outside." I thought then how much more apt a term it would have been for the Dakota settlers to use, being much more closed in, in a communications sense, than the Alaskans are, having no radio or television and not even telephones, at first. The *Sioux City Journal* was the paper we saw most commonly, and mail service was such that we received Monday's paper on Wednesday, if all went well and the roads and railroads were not blocked and we were able to get to the mailbox a mile and a half away. The *Journal* at that

time had a page in it once a week called the "Bingville Bugle."
As I recall, it was in the Tuesday paper, and it was a page none
of us ever missed reading, being the nearest thing to comics we
ever saw. It purported to be a weekly newspaper chronicling
the antics of the preposterous inhabitants of the preposterous
town of Bingville, illustrated with drawings. It was raucous
humor that any of us could understand, and it delighted us all.

The nights of the literary meetings were the rare ones, never
more than once a week, sometimes every other week, sometimes
omitted altogether on account of weather and roads. Most of our
winter evenings were spent at home, with no fretting on the
part of any of us about being bored or yearnings to seek entertainment on the outside, yearnings for the impossible being accepted as the height of futility. "Where shall we go tonight?"
was an unasked question. "What shall we do?" must find its
answer within our own walls.

Reading was always a part of the answer, when we had anything to read. Sometimes we did not, and there was never
enough. Finishing the last book we had borrowed from the
Smiths, and having it too stormy for several days to walk the
mile and a half to return it and get more, was a frequent and
painful experience. Seeing the end of my book approaching was
like eating the last bite of food on my plate, still hungry, and no
more food in sight.

Father made a checkerboard for us from the wooden end
of an orange crate, marking off the squares with ruler and
pencil. We used black and white buttons for checkers. We
made good use of orange crates for various purposes, such as
accessory pieces of furniture. They made acceptable book cases
and storage cabinets which could be tucked into very small
spaces. Not that we ever had a crate of oranges. Grocers used
them as containers for large orders of groceries bought by the
settlers.

The playing cards we were permitted to use one winter
afforded us much enjoyment, and it is painful to me in retrospect to think how much pleasure we sacrificed because of
puritannical fears. A Flinch deck, sent to us from relatives in
Iowa, was a welcome substitute for the playing cards. We literally wore out that Flinch deck. All the surface glaze was eroded
off the cards, and they seemed to get softer, thicker, and pulpier,
so that it was very difficult to shuffle them. In fact, one card
would scarcely slide against another, and they tore easily. They
were finally declared useless when many of the cards could be
identified as easily from the backs as from their faces, by the
tears on them.

The popcorn we popped on those winter evenings would have filled a silo, in the aggregate. For the seven of us, we needed enough to fill mother's largest dishpan. First, there was the shelling. Our popcorn did not come packaged. It had been planted in the field, hoed, the ripened ears picked and dried, at which stage they could be stored indefinitely, unless discovered by mice. The shelling was done by hand, by rubbing the thumb over the kernels to loosen them, or by rubbing two ears together. The thumb method, used for more than a few ears, could be wearing on the thumbs, as the kernels were very hard and tended to grow into sharpened points on the outer surface.

The dishful of fluffy popped corn could be treated in various ways, the usual one being with salt and melted butter. A fancier, more laborious preparation was the making of balls with the addition of sugar syrup or sorghum boiled to the right consistency. The aroma of the popped corn filled the house on these winter evenings. We munched happily as we pursued our various occupations—mother usually doing mending, while father, the boys, and I read or played Flinch or checkers, and the twins played with their dolls. Never was there popcorn left in the dishpan, except a few hard kernels; to be filled up on popcorn, not to be able to eat it all, was unheard of.

Candy making was another winter evening occupation greatly enjoyed but indulged in less often because of the cost. Using sugar for candy was an extravagance permissible only at Christmas. Sorghum was somewhat cheaper, and we always had several gallon pails of it among our winter food supply, so we made molasses taffy. Mother had charge of the boiling of the sorghum to the proper endpoint, then all the children participated in the rest of the process. First, hands had to be washed, no matter if they did not look dirty, as the boys and the twins sometimes protested. Then, with fingers lightly buttered, each of us picked up a small wad of the boiled and thickened molasses which had been set outside in the cold for a few minutes until cool enough to handle. From this point on, constant motion, agility, care, and watchfulness were called for. Mother did not do any of the pulling herself. She had her own hands full, supervising the rest of us, trying to minimize the amount that was dropped on the floor, stuck to clothing, or caught in somebody's hair. The proper procedure was to stretch the sticky mass as far as possible, bring it together again, stretch, twist, pull, and reassemble, over and over. As our efforts progressed, we could note changes in our product. The mass became firmer, offered more resistance to being pulled out, and was lighter in color. (The color change was more pronounced if mother had remembered to add a pinch of soda at the end of the boiling.) The final move of each of use was to stretch the mass one more time, to as even a circumference as possible throughout, give it several twists, and coil it on a buttered platter that mother had in readiness. The platter was then set outside in the cold again, for the coils of taffy to harden, which required only a few minutes. When Mother brought it in again, only a light tap with the back of the heavy butcher knife was required to break the coils into bite-sized pieces, shattering off splinters which flew all around the platter, in the process, which were immediately reached for by eager, grasping fingers, to mother's admonitions, "Now if you get your fingers in the way of my knife, you'll be sorry!" Other plates were ready for the serving of the flavorful bits, too hard to be bitten into—they must be sucked for quite an interval, until finally they could be chewed by sound, firm teeth, as exhilarating to the taste buds in one state as the other. (My mouth waters as I write.)

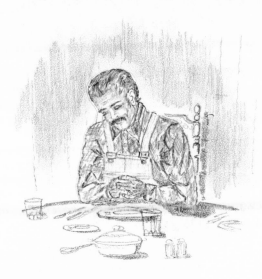

10 / PIONEER SPIRITUALITY

THE TRUE COLONIZER brings with him to the new land something more than his possessions and his personal ambitions. He sets up in his mind an ideal for the new country, seeing it as a utopian state having all the good features of the place from which he has come and none of its faults. His household established, his fields broken, his acres fenced and stocked—all this does not make a place home to him. The old lares and penates must be set in their accustomed places.

These are established as a matter of course, without conscious reasoning in their behalf. So far as the essentials of life were concerned, we lived much as we had always lived, maintaining the standards to which we were accustomed. We ate meals regularly and promptly, on the appointed hour. It was a lax housewife, according to father's thinking, whose family had to wait for its meals. It would have caused him acute embarrassment to bring his help to the house at noon and find dinner not in the actual process of being brought to the table. Each child was in his place, on the dot, with clean hands and face, and hair smooth. The menfolk used one comb in common. During the summer season it was kept in the "comb case" under the mirror, hanging on the outside of the house beside the door. Beneath it was the tin wash basin, on an upended orange crate, with the pail of water and a dipper beside it.

Grace was said before meals. Father always did this except when we had a male guest whom he thought it would not embarrass to be invited to say it. A white cloth covered the table; colored cloths were not the thing in those days among those who had any pride. We did own one red checkered cloth, used as a makeshift for wash day or housecleaning time, or on an occasional picnic.

We never wore ragged clothes just because there was no one to see what we wore. We always cleaned up for Sunday, both our house and our persons. There would always be a special Sunday dinner, with extra foods partly prepared the day before. Also, we observed the day as strictly as in the old days when there were people all about to observe what we did.

Father and mother were always quite rigid in their insistence upon the proper observation of the Sabbath. No ball games, picnicking, fishing, or hunting were allowed. Only the mildest diversions might be indulged in, such as a visit with friends or a walk or a drive. The idea of Sunday as a day of rest was so strictly ingrained in us that once when I had just learned a new crochet stitch I was so eager to proceed with it that in the secrecy of my room I crocheted nearly a half yard of the new lace on Sunday afternoon. Then, obsessed with guilt the next day, I unraveled it all. Mother, also, had a very prickly conscience in the matter of Sunday practices. In the former days in Iowa, on those occasions when we were having visiting relatives for Sunday dinner and mother stayed at home from church to cook, she always said the church bells rang louder and longer than usual that morning, and more than the usual number of people passed our house on their way to church.

We did not dance or play cards, these being Methodist taboos. A few of the settlers held barn dances occasionally—those few who had just built new barns with floors in them large enough to dance on—but we were never allowed to go. In this connection, I remember a little paperback book we had around home, *From the Ballroom to Hell*. For one winter there was a lapse in the strictness about cards for some reason. Father fell from grace to the extent of teaching us to play "High Five" and "Seven Up." We enjoyed playing, immensely, but I think father never felt just right about it, and mother disapproved from the first, being tortured by the fear of having her children grow up to be gamblers. So the cards disappeared before the next winter, and the games were never resumed in our house. We confined ourselves to Flinch and checkers.

Taking for granted the things we have always known—institutions, social privileges, gifts of progress—we quickly develop an appreciation of them when faced with their lack, and seek to reinstate them in our midst as soon as possible. Loving the strangeness of the new life, we nevertheless seek to erase it in all haste by substituting the old familiars as soon as possible. Thus many people in this Rosebud Country who had formerly regarded church as one of the take-it-or-leave-it graces of living, joined with the others in saying that of course we must have a church and Sunday school. The subject was broached one Saturday afternoon in Paxton when a group of settlers met by chance as they were doing their shopping.

"Wonder how long it will be before they get some kind of church services goin' around here. My wife's beginning to say she don't know as she wants to stay long in a country where they don't have church." The speaker thus adroitly pinned the responsibility for the notion on his wife, the appurtenances of religion being considered largely of feminine concern.

None of the other stalwart heads of families in the group appeared to see anything trivial in his suggestion, however, and they all gave it their attention. Apparently it had been a topic of discussion in the homes of all of them.

"Well, I guess 'they' means us," Herman Lebert volunteered. "I don't know as anybody is apt to start a church for us."

"Now I can't say as I've ever been a church-going man myself," George Dall said, "but I'll sure help support a church here. For my children's sakes, I wouldn't want this country to grow up without churches in it."

Thus the chance group became, then and there, a self-appointed committee to see that church services should be started in our community in another week. George Dall and John Evans promised to see about a meeting place that very afternoon, and the others would get the word spread around during the coming week.

Our first religious service was Sunday school, held in a dance hall in Paxton which seemed to be the only available building large enough. It had also the added advantage of a piano, one of the few in the area. It was played by Viola Cork, a talented hunchbacked girl who lived just over the line in Gregory County, and was therefore an "old settler," antedating us Tripp County people by several years. This first service was held on Sunday afternoon. Some families came six or eight miles, a long drive over the new roads, many of which were not yet roads at all but merely trails formed by a few who had gone before, picking the smoothest way. Lumber wagons were the commonest mode of conveyance, drawn by heavy work horses that were slow and plodding but the only horses most people owned as yet. A few had spring wagons, as we did. Others came on horseback. Every hitching post was taken that afternoon, and several had to tie their teams to the wagons of others. Paxton had the appearance of an unusually busy trading day.

At such a gathering, people's clothes mattered about as little as anyone could imagine. Anything that was clean and neat was considered acceptable. In fact, most people bought very few clothes of any sort during those first few years, except work clothes to replace those that wore out. Matters of fashion being cheerfully set aside by common consent, they wore out the clothes they had, regardless of vintage. When dressier clothes were finally unwearable, girls frequently wore calico to church, and the boys their newest pair of overalls.

Martin Schuler, a young man who had been a school superintendent in his old home, was elected superintendent of the Sunday school, and he made an earnest, capable one. His sister, Gertrude, who kept house for him while he lived on his claim, taught my Sunday school class. Having been a school man, Martin Schuler was more careful of his grammar than most of the settlers, and his comparatively good language set him apart from the rest with a certain amount of distinction. He was often addressed as "professor," a title synonymous in many people's minds with male teacher.

Each family brought any hymn books it possessed, and the oldest and most familiar hymns were chosen for singing, so that all might participate. Seating had been a question at the outset, one bound to be solved by a group so determined to have all the appurtenances of a religious service. Planks were finally borrowed from a building under construction, and laid across beer kegs lent by the saloonkeeper for the occasion. There was some dubiety and much jollity about the use of beer kegs in a place of worship, but the general opinion was that the sacredness of the purpose would hallow even a beer keg.

What earnest, religious, worshipful people this account makes us sound! After a week of hard work, to go to all this trouble and travel this distance to attend a religious service. It makes the church appear to have been very meaningful to us, as indeed it was. Honesty, however, compels me to record the other aspects of the case. For most of us, this service was the one break in a rather lonely week. It was going someplace after a week of staying at home, a time of social contacts after a week barren of them, talking to people outside one's own family, visiting with friends. In brief, we should have enjoyed this meeting, and made an effort to get to it, for whatever reason on earth it was being held. I even venture to guess it was the little gossipings and other friendly exchanges of a mundane nature which chiefly occupied our minds as we drove home rather than the Sunday school lesson. These factors should not be regarded as a detraction of religion, however, but merely an admission of human frailties.

We held religious services in the dance hall at Paxton just through the summer. By late fall a sod schoolhouse had been built just across the Tripp County line, about two miles west of Paxton, and church services were held there. A minister came out from Dallas on Sunday afternoon to preach to us. A significant fact in this connection is that I do not know what denomination he represented. He must have belonged to one of the orthodox, established denominations, as he had a charge in Dallas, but I do not recall that there was any discussion of his creeds. I think it quite likely he was a Methodist. Whatever religious doctrines swayed the preaching in this little sod schoolhouse, we all gathered there quite contentedly and complacently, finding no differences of opinion among us to make schisms in the group. Attending these services made quite a long drive for our family, but we went there to church throughout the first winter as regularly as the weather permitted. By the next year we had built a schoolhouse of our own, only a half-mile from where we lived.

Religious services in our own schoolhouse were conducted at irregular intervals by a series of itinerant ministers. We had church on the Sundays when a preacher was available. The one who came to us most frequently was old Mr. Campbell. He was a homesteader, too, several miles west of our neighborhood. We called him "old"—he was probably in his fifties, which was considerably older than the average of the homesteaders—and he had a full, flowing beard, which made him look to me like one of the ancient biblical patriarchs. He was a widower and lived all alone on his claim, doing his own cooking, of course, and all his other housework, including washing and ironing. The hardships he endured during the week, however, never reflected themselves in the disposition he showed to us on Sundays. He was a jolly, kindly, emotionally devout little man, without much refinement—a typical old-time Methodist, as we had known Methodist ministers in the small towns where we had lived. His rickety top buggy and his old white horse, Angelina, became a familiar and welcome figure in our neighborhood. The first time I met him he asked me promptly whether or not I was "saved." I replied hastily that I was, without knowing exactly what he meant, hoping at least to be thus "saved" from further such embarrassing questions.

Besides these sporadic Sunday services, one or more of the visiting preachers that came to us would occasionally organize a series of revival meetings held every evening for a period of a week or more. The settlers thronged faithfully to these meetings, filling all the seats, some of the men standing in groups around the stove in the back. Such a meeting gained in fervor as it progressed. There would be singing at first, old songs that everyone knew—"Stepping in the Light," "Jesus Saves," "Washed in the

Blood," "Just as I Am." Then there would be prayers, an impassioned sermon, and more singing. As the climax of the evening, the preacher would ask all those who felt themselves saved to come and occupy the front seats, the sinners remaining in the back. The object now was to glean some few more sheep each evening from this number that remained behind, the saved ones cooperating with the minister to this purpose. If some enraptured woman felt inspired to burst spontaneously into song or prayer, that was further evidence of the spirituality of the meeting, and the others appended hearty amens. Numbers of the saved ones appointed themselves emissaries to go out among the crowd and get others to "come forward." A row of trembling, sobbing, or singing derelicts-brought-to-port, kneeling at the altar at the close of the evening was evidence of a successful meeting. Where they would be a month or a year from that date, no one troubled about.

A session of "testimonies" was a regular part of the revival meetings, also, during which the more courageous arose and told the assembly of their own personal experiences in sin, and the victories of spirit over flesh. At their height, these sessions took on the nature of public confessionals. One evening when the crowd had been worked up to the hysteria of a "successful meeting," a young couple electrified the audience by confessing, in tears, that they had tasted of marital pleasures upon more than one occasion before their recent marriage. At that time, when sex was not recognized openly as existent, much less talked about, this young couple's disclosure was a real shocker. The preacher seemed quite nonplussed, having gotten, for once, more than he had bargained for.

Aside from their rather questionable moral value, it may be that these revival meetings bestowed benefits that have never been credited to them. One could not be saved, or have any assurance of a secure Christian standing, without losing himself in an emotional jumping-off place at some such religious "experience" meeting, which did give these too stolid, repressed, unsentimental people a vigorous loosening up, emotionally. Who knows that it may not have acted as a purge, also, of various unhealthful spiritual and mental debris? A thorough-going religious experience of this kind was the only type of hysteria allowable to sane and sensible people such as these.

Then, after a few weeks, these emotional debauches being over, the lives of the people resumed their normal trends—gin rummy, barn dances, and all. Who could imagine a wise and tolerant God finding offense in any of the simple pleasures of these people who asked for so little by way of diversion?

Thus was our spiritual life administered to, by fine, earnest, well-meaning, self-sacrificing clergy. They expounded the scriptures to us dogmatically, to the best of their enlightenment, stimulating our interest in the Bible, at least. They made articulate for us the ideals and virtues to which we aspired. They made us uncomfortable by vehement exhortations against the evils of drinking, smoking, card playing, and dancing, resulting for very short periods in rigorous vows of abstemiousness from such evils. When we fell from grace, some of the mentally nimble among us were able to exculpate ourselves by a transference of motive, as in the case of one good woman who told mother that she went to that barn dance just to see how silly and terrible it really was.

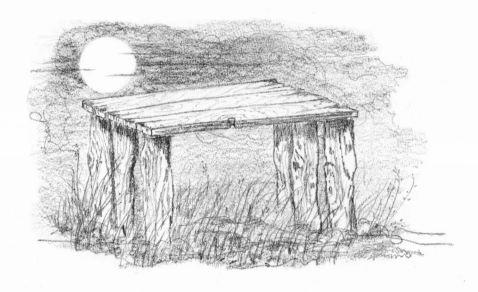

11 / HELPING UNCLE GRANT GET A FARM

WE KNEW FATHER was expecting some important mail when one day late in August he came in from the field an hour early and let Floyd ride Old Duke up to the mailbox. Our mailbox was on the Paxton road, a mile and a half north of our house. The mail came out from Paxton every weekday, but during the busy farm season or when the roads were blocked in winter we might not get to the mailbox for it more than twice a week.

Floyd and Duke were back at the house just at suppertime, Old Duke's gray coat darkened by streaks of sweat.

"What have I told you about riding those heavy work horses so hard?" father asked, sternly.

"But I couldn't hold him back, honest!" Floyd protested. "He wanted to trot all the way home!"

Old Duke hadn't had his supper, either.

Our meal that evening was fried prairie chicken. Father had taken his shotgun with him to the far pasture that morning, and brought home three plump young birds. They were in season now—not that it mattered. All the settlers ate them, in season and out. Out of season we referred to them as "prairie ducks," a species not mentioned in the game laws, or in any ornithology text. Game wardens were unknown to us, personally. Officialdom seldom penetrated this far from its offices. None of us went hunting for sport, anyway, only for a refreshing change from our ham and bacon meals.

Now, ecologists, do not point the finger of blame at us for having brought the prairie chicken to the point of extinction. We were in no wise to blame for that. We merely fitted ourselves into the natural laws of a country, by which one species feeds upon another for its livelihood. The only organized "hunts" I ever heard of there were those of the Langenfelder men when they rode out looking for jack rabbits and coyotes (and they never got many). If no one but the residents of Tripp County had ever shot its prairie chickens, their number would never have been depleted appreciably. Carloads and planeloads of hunters from Omaha, Des Moines, Chicago, and neighboring areas who vie with one another for numbers of game killed, are the exterminators of a species (and they are presently engaged in the extermination of pheasants in our area).

Father had read the letter he had been expecting. Now, when he had finished supper, he read it to us. It was from Uncle Grant, father's brother, saying he would be arriving within the coming week. Uncle Grant's full name was Ulysses Simpson Grant Cashatt, but I had heard father say that it would be worth a black eye or a bloody nose to anyone who called him that. Not that Uncle Grant was not a post hoc Union sympathizer, sure enough; but he was a modest, quiet man, much like father in that respect—not one to edge himself under a tent of glory erected over someone else.

Father's forebears had been farming people for as long as there was any record of them, and it was a disappointment to him that neither of his brothers had remained on the farm. He thought it indicated a flaw in their judgment, and his own temporary defection into the business world before we went to Dakota only strengthened this opinion. His older brother, Van, was a section foreman on the Milwaukee railroad, and Grant was a coal miner in Polk County, Iowa.

"And not very good coal, either," mother always commented when the subject came up.

So with squatters' day just a month away, father had written urgently to Uncle Grant not to miss this opportunity of getting a piece of land of his own at almost no cost. An opportunity that would never come again, as this Rosebud Country in South Dakota was the last land the government was likely to have to be offered on these terms.

Father didn't say he was glad Uncle Grant was coming, or anything like that. He was a taciturn man, not given to elaborating verbally on his own feelings. But he was whistling "Yankee Doodle" when he and the boys went out to do the evening milking, an unfailing sign that he was happy and lighthearted over something.

Visitors had not been at all uncommon throughout this first summer, considering our comparative isolation. They were usually men who had drawn numbers in the land lottery and were out looking for suitable quarter sections on which to file claim, or just looking over the situation in general, trying to decide whether to take the land at all. The settlers' jocular version of the governmental offer was, "The government bets you a hundred sixty acres of land against a thousand dollars that you can't live on it fourteen months without starving to death." Just a merry jest it was then, but a dozen years later, with the beginning of the drought and the scourges of grasshoppers, the jest had become a grim truth. Now, however, more and more of the brightly new little mushroom houses were springing up, men's outward pledge of faith in the South Dakota soil and the beneficence of Providence—thicker in the eastern part of the county near the Gregory County line, becoming sparser as one traveled westward.

As fall approached, these land seekers increased in number. The straggling little road that led past our claim became almost a thoroughfare. These strangers approached always from the north. That was the road that led out from Dallas, Gregory, and all the rest of civilization. Its only purpose in continuing south of us was to reach those few settlers more remotely situated than we were. Throughout September the boys watched the Dallas road daily for signs of visitors. They were a welcome interest and excitement to all of us.

"I see a team up on Smith's hill!" one of the boys would shout excitedly.

"And it isn't Mr. Fergen or Mr. Brumbaugh!" (our neighbors to the south) the other would add, as the vehicle approached closer. "So it must be a livery team."

Then if it were ten o'clock in the morning, or past that, they would rush in to tell mother that we would probably have company for dinner. Whereupon mother would admonish me to be sure to peel enough potatoes, and she would bustle about to see if there were not a little extra she might prepare for dessert. If there were no pie or cake in readiness she could always stir up a tasty cornstarch pudding, or a fruit something or other, often of her own invention. No matter what duties she had on hand for the day, I do not recall that she was ever cross on account of any extra work thus required of her, and not even those of her own intimate family circle were ever given cause to feel that such casual visitors were unwelcome.

Over the hills west of us there was quite a lot of unclaimed land. It was rougher country, having more of the jagged, rocky buttes, making it more picturesque, but less desirable for farming purposes. That range of hills is one of the indelible pictures in my memory. It think I must have looked at them every evening. The irregularity of their contours against the sky was interrupted in one place by a straight, slanting line, as though a slice had been taken out of it with a sharp knife. Any one of a medley of emotions may still transport me to them—sorrow, mental unrest, nostalgia, loneliness, or the fullest peace and contentment. Gazing upon them in the evening with the sun just gone behind them, I was able to grasp imageries and inspirations that I have never lost. It must be that the soul needs some such material focusing point. Sometimes I felt the sting of tears in my eyes, for no reason in the world that I could name except that the disappearing sun behind the hills seemed to symbolize everything that was tantalizing and unattainable. I have always had a very poor sense of direction, and to this day, whenever I wish to orient myself in strange surroundings, I automatically imagine myself facing those hills again, with my right hand to the north and my left hand to the south.

For those who had drawn numbers in the original land lottery, September 30 was the deadline. Land having no claim filed upon it by that time was open to squatter settlement, which was what Uncle Grant was contemplating. He arrived early in September, and he and father spent much time that month driving about looking at land. They finally decided upon a quarter section just a half-mile north of ours, as the most desirable one left available.

The law required that there must be no attempt to take possession of land by squatters' rights before midnight of September 30. At least that was the prevailing local understanding of the law. A man might travel all over the piece of land he was considering taking, up to the last day of September. On that final day, however, he was careful to keep entirely off it. Then the first man who made some "improvement" on the land after midnight of that crucial date, and filed his claim at the land office in Gregory, had priority of claim to the land title.

There was increasing excitement in the air as the end of the month approached. On the morning of the thirtieth father took Uncle Grant to the spot just off the piece of land that he wanted, and near the trail along which other land seekers would be driving, and left him there all day, sitting in or under the spring wagon. He brought the horses back home with him and went about his farm work for the rest of the day, and one of the boys went back on horseback at noon to take Uncle Grant his dinner. The purpose of all this was to make it plain to any wayfarer that he had chosen this particular quarter section upon which to file his claim, in the hope that others would then pass on to some other land rather than take their chances in a contest over this piece, which, of course, they would be apt to do. This was just an added precaution, for it was quite well known in any one neighborhood just who was planning to take up which piece of available land.

The boys and I were thrilled and delighted to the bubbling-over point when father told us that evening that we would be needed to help Uncle Grant get his claim. It made us feel very important to be involved, personally, in such an important piece of business. And how mad the twins were when they were told they were too little to go, and must stay at home and go to bed!

The chores were done early that evening, and we were ready to go by nine-thirty, but father insisted that ten o'clock was plenty early enough to start. The boys and I drove Duke and Barney hitched to the lumber wagon, in which were some posts, boards, hammer and nails, and a spade. Father and Uncle Grant had the lighter team, Gyp and Neil, with the spring wagon. That last day of September had been a scorcher. A whipping hot wind had blown all day long, keeping the prairie grasses continually bent before it, as though cringing and dispirited before this final blasting after a long summer of heat. Dakota nights, however, were nearly always cool, and there was a pleasant chill in the air as we set out. In the stillness all about us, it seemed that the creak of the wagon and the dull thud of the horses' hoofs in the sandy road might be carried for miles without being lost.

Father had put his shotgun in the spring wagon, telling mother jocularly that he might want to shoot at a jack rabbit if the moon were bright. But he did not fool mother; she knew there was too much else of interest at hand for him to bother about jack rabbits. She was quite uneasy about the whole expedition, and disapproved of having us children mixed up in it. We had all heard tales of wild and disastrous occurrences in connection with other squatters' nights. So father took his gun along, believing, as he did, in armed neutrality. We did hear shooting twice during the evening, somewhere to the west of us, and the next day we learned of several altercations, but none of a serious nature. The shooting we heard was doubtless celebratory in nature.

Our little cavalcade halted just off the border of Uncle Grant's intended property, with the team of sorrels headed down the trail toward Gregory. Father sat with his watch in his hand, and promptly a minute after midnight we drove across the border and unloaded the building materials we had brought. We had a lantern, too, but the moon was so bright we did not need to use it. It required about fifteen minutes to erect this particular "improvement" which the government required as a symbol of good faith and actual homesteading intentions. It was the homemaking motive the government encouraged, not the grabbing of land for financial profit. The posts were set shallowly in the ground and the boards nailed across the tops of them to hold them up. This, then, was the first "building" on Uncle Grant's claim. Fortunately, the government did not require it be given a name.

Then father and Uncle Grant drove to Gregory with the light team, leaving us to take Duke and Barney and the heavy wagon home. They were in Gregory when the land office opened, but they had to wait their turn, as the town was full of squatters, so it was late afternoon when they reached home again. The aptness of the expression "doing a land office business" occurs to me in this connection, and suggests its origin.

The next morning when we had the chores and housework done, mother suggested that we take a drive about the countryside to see what changes might have come about during the night, so the boys hitched Duke and Barney to the wagon again and we set out. Mrs. Evans and her two boys, Ward and Earl, from near Paxton, were on a similar exploring trip and had stopped at our house, so they went with us. John Evans, her husband, had gone to Gregory with a squatter friend of his own whom he was helping to get located.

We drove west, since most of the vacant land lay in that direction. A jaunt across virgin prairie in a lumber wagon is a slow, plodding trip, with elements of surprise, even of hazard, in it. We picked our way around the sharp buttes, up the gentlest slope of a ridge, along a creek for some distance, at times, before we found a place to cross without too much danger of tipping over. In the matter of picking a route, Duke and Barney themselves had fully as much judgment as any of the rest of us. Even on the apparently level stretches the prairie gave a decidedly humpy sensation upon being traversed with wheels. This was especially true when there were patches of a kind of fine grass that formed a dense, wiry network of roots, very difficult to cut or break, and not at all springy to ride over. Prairie dog towns, too, had to be avoided, lest a horse step suddenly into one of their holes and break a leg.

Just over the nearest range of hills we found the first evidence of squatter occupancy, a triangular shelter with a roof boarded over the top of it with pieces of packing boxes. There were a kerosene stove and some cooking utensils sitting under it. This proved to be a very transient abode, and disappeared after a week, the squatter apparently having lost faith in his venture. Perhaps he was wise, or perhaps he lacked vision. In either event, he apparently failed to see any promise of security in the face of the prairie about him. It may be that the thought of blizzards that would be sweeping through the gap in the hills there in the northwest in a few months struck terror to his heart and he returned to some place where he would have companionship, at least, against the buffetings of the world of nature.

We described a circle in our journey, angling off southwest from this point, then north again, and east. We found several other squatters' settlements, all of the same flimsy, temporary structure, intended only as gestures of tenancy. Some of these were ludicrous in their originality. One was a partly dug storm cave with a tent pitched nearby, in which a woman and two small children awaited the return of the father. The mother was somewhat frightened at our approach, disclosing the fact that fear lay not far below the surface of whatever thrill this adventure held for her. Here she was, destined to sit and wait, feeling herself quite defenseless against any danger that might threaten, encumbered with two children too small to walk any great distance, and having no mode of conveyance to any place of greater safety. Her relief when we stopped to talk to her and told her that we were neighbors from just a couple of miles over the hills, was pathetic.

"O, I'm so glad to know there are people that close!" she told us, with fervent thankfulness. Apparently in her own mind she was measuring her aloneness by the appearance of the prairie about her, and felt it to be limitless. Here, we felt, was just another variety of the courage that goes into the building of a frontier.

Winding our way now toward home, we came to another new structure that was occupied. It consisted of four stakes driven into the ground, each about three feet high, with a piece of an old bed blanket stretched over the top of them. Under this canopy a Plymouth Rock hen was tied by one leg to one of the stakes. She was scuttling about busily within the limits of her tether, catching the occasional grasshopper that became available; finding this apparently a happy hunting ground, where grasshoppers were ingenuous creatures with no experience in dodging hens. Her absent owner had provided amply for her with a pan of water and some shelled corn scattered about. We could not imagine how she had escaped the notice of the coyotes for this long, unless it was that the coyotes, being wild prairie creatures, were not yet trained to look for their food in shelters.

Coyotes were plentiful in this country. We saw them frequently, but never very close by. Our usual sight of them was of a brownish, bushy-tailed animal, somewhat smaller than a collie dog, galloping in the opposite direction, looking warily over his shoulder as he went. A coyote's howling is a sound one remembers. I never heard one making a halfhearted sound of any kind. They always wail in utter abandonment, and to the inexperienced ear one coyote can sound like a whole pack of them. We heard them every evening in the summer, usually at dusk. I suppose they really do howl for the same reasons that other animals make sounds—to communicate with their fellows, attract mates, and so on, but they sound like nothing so much as a despair encompassing all eternity.

Uncle Grant's interest in his land-holding project had been just luke-warmish at first, but by the time he had returned from Gregory where he saw so much enthusiasm, he had succumbed to the infectiousness of the land craze, and he became as wholehearted in his purpose as any of the others. He went back to Des Moines a few days later to get Aunt Susie—they had no children—and the two of them stayed with us while he was building his house.

Uncle Grant's house was unique, different from any other we had ever seen. It was a half-dugout. Into a steep hill on the east boundary of his land he dug quite a roomy chamber; then he built the projecting front part of sod. In this front wall were two windows and a door. The floor was made of wide pine boards, and the walls were plastered neatly on the inside. It was the warmest type of prairie home, a burrow into the very bosom of the earth. There could be no drafts under the floor here, and the Dakota blizzards could only sweep impotently over it. The swirling snow could block the door and windows, and frequently did, but could not penetrate the snugness inside. On such occasions an alabaster tunnel, deep as a man's height, had to be dug for egress. The boys and I loved to visit Uncle Grant and Aunt Susie, and considered a floundering walk through the snowdrifts and cold well rewarded when we walked through the welcoming tunnel to the door and the cozy hospitality inside.

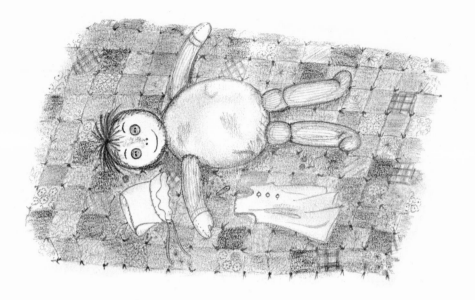

12 / TORTURINGS AND FRUSTRATIONS

IT IS WORTHY OF NOTE that the chronicler of a pioneer age is apt
to set down with gusto, sometimes even with some exaggeration,
I suspect, the physical rigors endured. This, it is said, is evidence of the superior stamina of the people of that time. "How
tough we were; how strong! No weaklings, we!" Whereas the
abrasions of the spirit come less readily to the surface of the
mind for voluble release, being more painful to recall, and possibly more telltale in their interpretations.

The fact of proximity itself is a sufficient cause for some
disharmony among seven people living in two small rooms. Evidence of strain in our parents, which we children did not understand, became very upsetting to us at times causing us to wonder
fruitlessly what mother was crying about; why father was so
cross. In retrospect, the comparative equanimity they were able
to maintain seems remarkable in the face of all the risks, uncer-
tainties, frustrations, worries, and the grilling toil that came to
be the prominent pattern in their days.

As we accumulated more and more livestock, the possibilities for disaster increased and became more variegated. Our first
two milk cows, lonely for others of their kind and perhaps suffering from sexual frustrations, were continually running away.
Fencing, tethering, elaborate yokes designed to hamper their
agility, were only temporary discouragements, equally futile in

the end. "Looking for the cows" became a disheartening and oft-repeated journey, usually on foot, sometimes on horseback. They could almost be trusted to run away whenever father was gone for a few days on a business trip. Father's absences were also the occasions for a pig to die, a horse to get cut in the barbed wire fence, or a coyote raid on the chickens.

Being a long way from a doctor must have caused the settlers some perturbation at times, but it was seldom spoken of. They were not expecting to get sick. One alarming episode in our family was Marie's convulsion at the onset of a sore throat with a high fever. The doctor from Dallas arrived some hours later, and left her some medicine. Kindly Mrs. Smith suffered the worst complication of Marie's illness. Trying to be of help to mother, she had pried Marie's mouth open with her finger to get her to take her medicine, and was bitten by the recalcitrant patient.

Father's attack of severe, low, right-sided abdominal pain was an illness of possible more serious import. After the long, jolting ride to Dallas in the lumber wagon, the doctor diagnosed his trouble as acute appendicitis and advised him to have an appendectomy. The nearest surgeon, and the nearest hospital, were fifty-odd miles farther east, and father knew nothing about either of them, so he elected to go back home and treat himself with Chamberlain's Pain Relief, a drug store medicament in alcoholic solution which produced a pleasant warm glow in the stomach after swallowing. Risky as his decision was, he felt there were more risks in the alternative open to him, and he may have been right. Right or wrong, luck was with him. He recovered quite promptly. Many years later he had an abdominal operation which confirmed the Dallas doctor's diagnosis; his appendix was reported hardened and shriveled from an old infection.

A minor but almost constant source of discord in our family was the running feud between the boys and the twins. "Make them stop picking on us!" the twins wailed frequently to mother, making it necessary for her to inquire into the provocations which were seldom difficult to establish. The most heinous of these arose from the habit the twins had of sitting on the boys' bed in the daytime to sew their doll clothes, this being a nice sociable spot near where mother was working. But they were impulsive, distractible little creatures, and when they were finished with their sewing they often neglected to remove the pins and needles they had stuck in the boys' pillows while they were working.

In general, these dolls of the twins were almost unendurable to the boys. Floyd and Fern both detested them, made fun of them, practiced indignities upon them, would have immolated them except for fear of parental reprisals. These dolls were, indeed, anything but beautiful. They were rag dolls that mother had made for them by cutting the figures from some worn-out sheets, stuffing them with cotton, and drawing the facial features with a pencil. They were handled so much that they became as dirty as any badly soiled garment, and needed frequent washing which eventually obliterated the features so that they had to be redrawn. Finally the cloth would wear through and leave the cotton stuffing sticking out, so that the faces and parts of the bodies would have to be replaced, and so on. They were as nearly immortal as any dolls ever were. They were security symbols, I realize now, and I think the boys sensed that without understanding it. They knew there was something that gave those pesky twins the stamina to stand up against them, and they blamed the dolls more rightly than they knew.

The names the twins gave their dolls infuriated the boys almost as much as the dolls themselves. For some weird reason none of us could understand, they called them "Halley" and "Larson." Halley's Comet was still fresh in our memories, and we had known numerous Larsons, but what strange sense of euphony suggested these as fitting names for dolls remained an enigma. We all tried to talk them out of it, but to no avail. "Make the twins name their dolls something decent!" Floyd plead agonizingly to mother, but by this time the depth of his concern had begun to seem ridiculous to her, and she could only laugh at him. The most daring attack the boys ever made on Halley and Larson was to bury them in a strawstack behind the barn. But whatever ill happened to the dolls, there was never any question who the culprits were, and they were speedily brought to terms. The penchant of the twins for bizarre names was not limited to their dolls. In some of their secret dream-world games they christened mother "Teed," and continued to call her that for several years. This was fully as enigmatical to the rest of us, and almost as infuriating to the boys as their naming of their dolls, to which mother, wisely, paid little heed.

The severest disruption of our peace of mind in these Dakota days was corporeally the smallest enemy we ever had to deal with. Whenever I see an exterminating company's vehicle on the street, I think what a boon such a service would have been to the Dakota settlers. Mass exterminations were unknown in those days. They were an individual or a family matter, carried out painstakingly by hand. There were no discriminating sprays that would destroy the parasite and leave the host in good health. Potato beetles had to be picked or shaken off each plant into a container and then disposed of, usually by burning; the horrendous tobacco worm that sometimes infested our tomato plants, too immense to be thought of as a mere larval form, was usually pried off the foliage with two sticks and then chopped to death with a hoe; the fleas on the hounds were usually a matter of canine endurance and survival.

Other exterminations imposed the added burden of secrecy. For these there was not the comfort of neighborly sympathy and counsel. Every family's struggle was its own isolated warfare, a disheartening undercover battle without assistance from allies. For whom could one trust with such a secret? We were all new people, shucked out of our backgrounds and set down in a strange country, stripped of the sheltering vestments of tradition. Face values were the only judgments our neighbors had to go by. Whatever reputations we had had for honesty, cleanliness, decency, were unknown here, and had to be built up anew, which takes time. We could not risk being pigeon-holed in the minds of strangers as "the family that has bedbugs."

I wonder now that it did not occur to us sooner that if such a scourge could descend upon us out of this clean and virgin prairie, it could be descending likewise upon the rest of the settlers. But we were so stricken at first that it was a long time before we could lift our thoughts above our own humiliation and our frantic efforts to deal with it in a practical way. I think mother's first suspicion that we were not the only ones suffering this secret shame was aroused by a remark made by the itinerant preacher, Mr. Campbell, on one of his early visits to us. He had told us that he lived alone. "But," he added cryptically, "if that shack of mine ever burns down, there will be a terrible loss of life."

Other confirming data gradually came to light. Once we saw wooden bedsteads, springs, and mattresses strewn on the grass in front of a settler's shack, as happened with such painful periodicity at our house in our efforts at eradication of our infestation. Sitting in church one Sunday, Floyd nudged mother and pointed gleefully to one of the little brown vermin crawling on the coat collar of a man sitting in front of us.

There were agonizing speculations in family council as to the origin of our scourge. Mother said that maybe they were in the prairie grass, but father scoffed at this. She never saw any out there, did she? "In the lumber" was another suggested source, not given much credence. "If only I had known something about them before we came, and had been on the lookout for them!" mother reiterated, over and over. Years afterward, when the battle was over and the settlers could feel decent and complacent about it all, and could philosophize among themselves, I think they decided that the blame lay in old infested freight cars in which our goods had been shipped. If so, a blight on any of the officials of the Northwestern Railroad that were knowingly guilty!

Our family was probably the most severely afflicted of any of the settlers, owing to a piece of coincidental misfortune—the necessity for moving our house, after it was all finished and plastered, to another corner of our land where we could obtain a better water supply. Father had said that he would fix the plaster late in the fall, after the crops were in. This was the busy season, during which all the long daylight hours must be spent in attending to the crops. It seemed reasonable to all of us that repairs to our walls might wait until the rush was over. If they could be made in time to protect us from the cold of the winter, that would be soon enough.

Little did we know how accurately we were playing into the hands of a then unsuspected enemy! For by that time the genus *Cimex* probably had its colonization plans well organized, ready to take advantage of any break that offered itself; and here was a "break" in our plaster, like a mountain pass, making accessible to them fastnesses beyond the reach of any forces that could be brought to bear against them. So secure was their stronghold that they learned to depend upon no other shelter. And so unrelenting was mother's vigilance against them that the name *Cimex lectularius* was hardly descriptive of our particular visitation. They were, more strictly speaking, *Cimex muralis*.

The torturing awareness of their mass entrenchment behind this unassailable parallel we thought marked the end point of endurance for all of us. But upon mother, at least, a few comparatively small bands of them were to inflict a still keener suffering. When she found that they had infiltrated the few pitiful treasures of our cultural life, she terrified us children by demanding of father that he burn the house down.

It happened one rainy evening when we were wanting something new to read. Mother pulled a box of books from under one of the beds, where books that were supposedly too old for us were kept until we should have grown into them. This evening she took out *Scottish Chiefs*. It was a tattered volume that would have been considered worn out by any decent library standards, having barely survived the reading appetite of her own childhood and that of her brothers and sisters. Many pages were loose, and the scraggly cover had been reinforced with a piece of oilcloth. I remember her smile of pleasant reminiscence as she lifted it gently from the box, and the horror-stunned rigidity of her face as she peered beneath the cover to adjust a wrinkle in the oilcloth. None of us asked what she had seen. We knew.

For a long time no one moved, or said anything. Mother sat in an attitude of chilled abstraction, the book still in her hands. Then she laid it quietly back in the box, arose, and took down a picture that hung on the wall. It was a water color from Paris that someone had sent her as a wedding present. We all cherished this picture. For us children, especially, it had a very romantic association, as no one we knew had ever been to Paris. It was a pretty picture, too, a pleasant little autumn scene painted somewhere along the Left Bank.

The premonition that had led mother to take down the picture told the rest of us what she would find when she looked under the edges of the paper pasted across the back. After one despairing glance she set the picture on the floor against the wall, threw herself down on the sanitary couch that was the boys' bed at night, and gave way to the only attack of hysteria I ever knew her to have.

In this emergency father, calm as always, marshaled all his talents for logic and poise. He did not deny that mother's wild demand that the house be burned would destroy the enemy. "But it would be a pretty extravagant victory," he countered. "With some planning and patience, we can get rid of them without such a sacrifice on our part. And we'll set about it very soon."

This simple and positive declaration by father set things right for mother very promptly. I think she had imagined, heretofore, that our scourge was sitting too lightly upon him; whereas he was only waiting for the optimum time to take action against it. She should have known that he was not a man to tolerate living under such conditions any longer than necessary.

The time for action came within a few weeks, a more sweeping one than mother had dared hope for. After the last of the corn was picked, father delighted mother by telling her that there would be time before the stormy weather of winter to build on the extra room that we needed so badly. It was only a lean-to ell on the main part of the house, which was divided into a room for the boys and the kitchen, but it gave us a feeling of luxury to be able to reserve the rest of the house for a living room and two more bedrooms. Most important of all, the damaged plaster was repaired, the defective joinings in the woodwork were sealed up tight, thus imprisoning the guerrilla bands of *Cimex* ensconced in the walls.

The blockade held. By spring, mother was able to laugh a little over the whole affair.

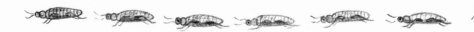

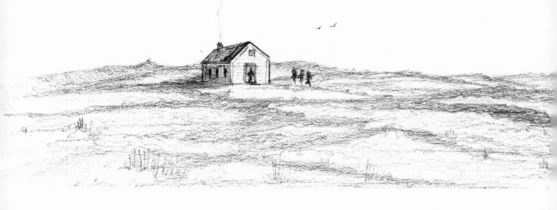

13 / FIRST SCHOOL

SCHOOLS were one of the urgent and immediate concerns of Dakota's new populace, next to be considered after the necessities of housing and food. Most of the settlers were people in their prime, with a number of children of school age. Those whose children were already grown were greatly in the minority and they were seldom the ones who were aspiring to the deeds to the new land. These were apt to be men like Mr. Fergen, to the south of us, who had come only to assist his daughter in her homesteading venture. Pioneering is, indeed, young people's work, and not only for physical reasons on account of the hardships that must be endured; minds must not be too set and formed. They must be pliable enough for all the plannings, innovations, dreamings, imaginings, that pioneering calls for, and strong enough to bear the frustrations and disappointments.

The soddy I have mentioned, just across the line in Gregory County, was the first schoolhouse built in our vicinity. Martin Schuler, the "professor" who was our Sunday school superintendent, was also the first teacher in this school. There was some talk of sending us there, but it was six miles away, and we could not have attended at all regularly in stormy weather. There was too much likelihood that the roads might be blocked for weeks at a time. So, several months later, our own little frame schoolhouse was built on the southwest corner of Uncle Grant's claim. It was called Sunnyside as it was situated on the south side of a hill, or perhaps because most of the settlers had known a Sunnyside where they came from.

At the time of the consolidation of schools throughout the Midwest, and the abandonment of these small country schoolhouses, much adverse comment was heard about them. It became an almost universally expressed opinion, "How drab that

100

little country schoolhouse looks! I wouldn't send my children to a place like that for anything! I should think it would be positively depressing to a child."

But how different things can seem in the eyes of a child! To me the school was a delightfully separate little world where one might have unfolded to him wonders he had never dreamed of and which he would never find anywhere else. There was so little provided for us to work with that we had to draw upon all our natural resources including our imaginations. Our playground was a sandy yard from which the prairie grass was soon worn off in scraggly patches. With sticks, stones, piles of brush, and scratched lines on the ground we made houses, bases for dare base and baseball, goals, prisons, Indian Country, or whatever else we needed to equip the current fantasy. We made most of our own baseballs by wadding tightly some soft material—old stockings were good for this—and winding it firmly with all the string we could save.

Twenty-three of us were enrolled in the first school term at Sunnyside, in all the grades from the first to the eighth, inclusive. Some hasty arithmetic would indicate there was not time enough for that many classes in the six hours of academic sessions. That rigorous schedule was encompassed, however, and was the accepted routine for rural schools of that day. Types of enrollment in individual schools suggested ways to manage. Small classes could often be combined, and study periods, of course, coincided with recitation periods in other classes.

The proverbial troublemakers in rural schools of that day were the big boys who were apt to dissipate their surplus energies in pranks and general rambunctiousness. Organized athletics for healthy workouts was nonexistent. Helping with the chores mornings and evenings at home was not always enough to keep them worn down sufficiently. Then, too, many of them saw their school careers coming to an end with the eighth grade, if not before. They would be working steadily forever after, and this was their last chance to have some fun with any kind of gang.

The problem pupil in this school, however, was Myrie, a lank, gangly girl of fifteen. She was supposed to be taking the seventh grade, but her mental capacities would have been strained to do work of fourth grade caliber. She was strong and athletic and could run like an ostrich. She was singled out for baiting by the other children, as such people frequently are, and she rose to it in a manner to fill her vandal tormentors with mixed delight and terror. She would tackle any of them, or all of them at once, and they could find no safety in flight since she could outrun any of them.

Myrie's personality, however, had begun to undergo a change. At intervals she made an attempt to be less hoydenish, apparently realizing that she was now a young lady. A part of this was an awakening of her sex consciousness. She began to take an interest in boys aside from her appreciation that they were nice to fight with. She paid attention to clothes for the first time, and achieved some rather fantastic effects by way of jabots, sashes, ribbons, and jewelry, while her free-swinging braids of hair were transformed to a mass of frizzes.

These changes in Myrie were discomfiting to some of her male schoolmates. They enjoyed the challenge in defending themselves from her in physical combat, but her amorous advances routed them. A neighbor boy, Harry, was her preference. She would watch for Harry to pass her house on his way to school, then she would set out to catch him and walk to school with him. She could do this easily since there was no running away from her. Then poor Harry would be tortured for the rest of the day by the gibes of his schoolmates. The situation was acutely painful to him, but he finally devised a scheme to circumvent it. He would pass Myrie's house, as usual, hide in the cornfield by the roadside until she had passed him in her pursuit, then crawl out of hiding and proceed in solitary comfort.

Myrie's amorous life, from that time on, was a succession of unreciprocated crushes on youths with whom she became acquainted, including the coach in the Dallas High School which she attended for a year. Finally she married a local youth of her own mental caliber, and immortalized all her previous passions by naming a succession of sons for the various objects of her affections, in turn. Perhaps a more healthful and sensible a procedure, at that, than the repression psychoses of other women with similar disappointments.

The first teacher at Sunnyside was Edie Sanders, daughter of an old-timer in Gregory County. She did not have a teacher's certificate, but was hired tentatively, pending the results of the examination to be given in Winner, two months hence. She entered blithely on her job, hoping that this time she would make a passing grade on the exams and be allowed to continue, although she had failed on three previous occasions.

Edie boarded with a Holland family in the neighborhood, the Van der Tuins, and hoped to use her time after school in studying for the tests. It was a difficult job, fitting this group of youngsters who had been out of school for awhile and had tasted the joys of running wild, into an orderly, scholarly curriculum, and she was totally inadequate for it. I think it was not scholastic training that she lacked, but an I.Q. that would never permit her to attain it. She made some attempts to study in the evenings to prepare herself for the exams, but her powers of concentration were very poor. Old Mr. Van der Tuin who was spending some months with his son, said of her, "She read and read, and she hear all our talk at the same time; vot is not right. Ven my boy Schon read a book, I say to him 'Schon! Schon!,' and he hear nottings."

Those were a hectic few months for poor Edie. There was mischief about all the time—giggling, pranks, and practical jokes of all kinds—and so much noise and confusion it would have been impossible for a conscientious pupil to study unless he possessed extraordinary powers of concentration. There was a parody on "Put on Your Old Gray Bonnet," which we made applicable to Edie, and never tired of singing or humming. It had its inspiration in a furry winter hood that she wore.

Edie would remonstrate with the mischief makers, scold, threaten, pout, and then burst out laughing at some of their nonsense. She had one means of retaliation which seemed to be a source of great comfort to her, and she used it with a vengeance. When she made out our report cards she gave us grades in deportment which, if they were as soothing to her ruffled spirits as they were startling to parental eyes, must have made our scores about even. It never occurred to her that failing grades in deportment in the majority of her pupils might in themselves constitute an indictment of her teaching prowess.

At our house, these grades very nearly resulted in our being taken out of school. Mother reasoned that if the teacher at school could not see that we spent our time to some profit, she might better see what she could do for us at home. It was only with much cajolery and solemn promising that we were allowed to continue.

Considering the trouble she was having, I think it was as much a relief as anything else to Edie when she learned that she had failed for the fourth time to pass the examinations, and that it would be necessary for her to give up her teaching career. She was married not long after this, and we heard she made a much better housekeeper than teacher. Her harrowing experience at Sunnyside must have netted her enough to buy some of her household furnishings, for the school board gallantly assumed upon the district the burden of their blunder in having hired her, and paid her full salary without quibbling.

Edie's job was now taken over by Jim Burchett, a lean, handsome, square-jawed young man who lived with his wife and two little girls on a homestead three miles east of the schoolhouse. He was bright, earnest, and well qualified, and had had some previous teaching experience. He was a rigid disciplinarian, the more rigid, perhaps, because of the dubious reputation the school had already attained. He started out with the idea that someone would be trying to make trouble for him, and was continually on the alert for it. He walked to school every morning, a graceful, athletic figure, swinging along with great strides, wearing a short jacket and a coonskin cap; carrying his lunch box under one arm and usually some books under the other.

He was an excellent teacher in most ways, but exceedingly didactic. Free and easy reading with natural expression was not enough for him. The punctuation marks were stop and go signs to be observed strictly. The reader must drop his voice with a decided thump at a period, pause briefly at a comma, a little longer at a semicolon, and so on. He was known to spend an entire class session drilling some frightened pupil whose voice persisted in rising instead of falling at the appropriate place. He drilled us mercilessly in accuracy of detail in many other things as well. For him everything must be done with almost mathematical precision.

Jim Burchett had a number of talents. He sang well, and made the "opening exercises" quite enjoyable, tuneful sessions. He wrote a beautiful hand, and did what we thought was excellent freehand drawing. He would draw seasonal pictures on the blackboard for us, with colored chalk, and when one of these pictures was in progress we would often stay in from recess and watch its development in fascinated wonder. No one but a real artist, we were convinced, could draw anything like that, and we considered him quite a marvel.

In one drawing he made, illustrative of the fall season, he drew a border of purple grapes across the top of the blackboard, and a variety of vegetables beneath it. When he had finished drawing a pumpkin he stopped and asked us what it was. "A punkin" came a chorus of replies, and, pinpointing the pupils in turn, he failed to find anyone who pronounced it otherwise. So throughout the rest of the week we were drilled on that word, until most of us remembered to say it properly—inside the schoolroom. Not the bravest of us would have dared to call it anything but "punkin" in ordinary conversation. It would have been considered a silly affectation, and we should have been hooted at. One boy even changed the pumpkin pie to mince, in a Thanksgiving story he had to write for his language lesson, because he said he felt so foolish saying it that way.

A short story written by another boy in language class illustrated the strictures in Mr. Burchett's training. This boy led his free-swinging characters through a number of adventures, and then faced a dilemma. How dispose of them and end the story? The tidiness he had had inculcated in him did not permit him to slide off his paper, leaving their destinies unresolved. So in one final paragraph, in one brief sentence after another, he recorded the demise of each of them.

Mr. Burchett had a few disciplinary problems, the most daring of which involved Floyd, the two Custer boys, and Emil Bush. From the day he started to school, Floyd had been a mischievous nuisance to his teachers at times. He and these other boys finally became restive under Mr. Burchett's strict methods and planned a revolt. Floyd was to start things by replying impudently when asked about an overdue geography paper. When Mr. Burchett reacted vigorously to this baiting, as he could be depended upon to do, the Custer boys and Emil were to come to Floyd's assistance and the four of them would give him a sound trouncing. Floyd made the impudent reply, as was planned, but when Mr. Burchett had him by the collar in a firm grasp, and Floyd looked about for the promised assistance from his three aides, they were studying away as though their lives depended upon it, apparently oblivious to the trouble he had gotten himself into. The affair ended in Floyd's being expelled from school for a brief period, a thorough talking over of things a short time later, and a firm and lasting friendship between him and Mr. Burchett afterward.

A concomitant of rural schooldom was the dinner pail, one of the least nostalgic of my memories in that connection. It was no fancy lunch box, with trick vacuum bottle insert, and so on, but a lard or syrup pail; a half-gallon size for one person, a gallon size for several. We always preferred to take individual lunches, but that was a luxury Mother was not much in favor of, as it meant five dinner pails to be scrubbed out each evening and well aired for the next day, so usually she reduced the number to two, or three at the most. Sometimes, for brief intervals, we carried our lunches in wooden grape baskets, and felt that these were quite fancy, but they were not strong enough to stand for long the rough usage to which they were subjected.

The enjoyment of these school lunches had to be sharply whetted by hunger, for they were anything but palatable in their own right. The flavor of sandwiches is not improved by remaining packed tightly in a pail for a half day, even if the glass of fruit sauce or preserves has not been spilled over them by the swinging of said pail on the way to school, or by its having been kicked over in the rumpus by someone attendant upon the removing of wraps and overshoes. Cookies so closely packed go through a peculiar softening process, making them altogether·

different from the crunchy discs which Mother had baked. The apple, if any, was probably eaten at recess.

Other children's food usually looked more attractive than one's own, and there was a universal bartering of lunches. Sometimes a group of us would picnic together, laying out all the food on one desk, or on the shady side of the schoolhouse when the weather was agreeable. We liked to trade edibles with the Van der Tuins. They had many cookies, coffee cakes, and other baked delicacies, made after Holland recipes that were new to us. We found these sweets to be very tasty.

One family of children often brought fried egg sandwiches, with the eggs fried soft, which gave a messy, drippy effect on faces, clothing, desks, sometimes even on the floor. These sandwiches were not much in demand for trades. The liquid part of our lunch was cold water carried in a pail from a well a half-mile down the hill, and drunk from a common dipper. Our occasional colds and sore throats were thus passed about freely from mouth to mouth, but they were caused by our own private community strains of organisms, to which we eventually developed some immunity. Our isolation protected us from most new and more virulent infections, so that the incidence of illness among us was not high.

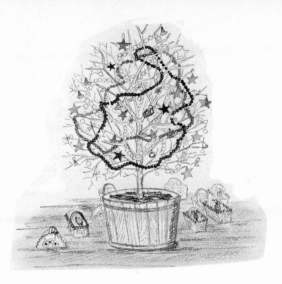

14 / THE GLORY TREE

ONE TEACHER we had at Sunnyside was a charming young woman who has remained linked in my mind inseparably with the Christmas celebration she arranged for us that year. I see her now as she stood before us beside her desk, a slender figure in a white shirtwaist and a black skirt that reached almost to her ankles, her hair a shiny, smooth cap with a coil on each side of her head, her face radiant with planned joys for her beloved pupils sitting expectantly in front of her.

She wore her watch half-way down the front of her shirtwaist, hung by a chain around her neck. The lid opened noiselessly when she pressed the stem, but it closed with an authoritative snap that could be heard all over the schoolroom. She seldom looked at her watch except at the close of a fifteen-minute class period, and she seemed to know when that was, before looking. It was just a part of the closing routine. In the same way that a modern school might use electric bells, the closing of teacher's watch clicked forward another cog in the day's schedule.

But the watch made another sound sometimes—a soft, muted meshing of the thin gold lid, which was only faintly audible. I never could determine exactly what made this changed sound, but she seemed to be holding the watch cupped more closely, even lovingly, in her hand at these times. Perhaps we only imagined this change of sound, seeing in her pretty face the benign look of a contemplated happiness for a roomful of children. For just as the click signaled the end of a usual class period, this soft watch sound meant some pleasant variation in the day's routine.

107

Hearing it now, in this after-recess final quarter of the school day, we awaited with alert expectancy whatever it was that teacher had in mind. Pencils were laid down, papers stopped rustling, my seatmate closed her history book and put it back in the desk. Teacher corroborated our hopeful anticipation by standing quietly for a few moments, prolonging the delightful suspense. On ordinary days she would already be unrolling the map for seventh-grade geography class.

Coming, as this did, on Monday of the second week of December, we guessed that teacher's plan had something to do with Christmas. Most things we did these days had Christmas woven into them. When teacher would ask, "What shall we do for opening exercises this morning?" there would be a flurry of excitedly waving hands. And whichever child she called upon, his request was apt to be, "Let's talk about Christmas," or "Let's sing some Christmas songs."

We all loved this, even we three older ones, who liked to consider ourselves past childish delights. Teacher loved it too, and this feeling of hers made warm and personal the stories of the Christ child, the wise men, Bethlehem, and the star. And the singing!—for the talking was always interspersed with a Christmas song or two. Our school had an organ, which many schools did not have, and when teacher sat down and played "Silent Night" we felt rich with happiness and tingled with it as we sang.

Some of the talk would be about Christmas legends, family customs, and celebrations of the Holy Day in other lands. Teacher told us many stories her mother had told her about the old-time festivities in Sweden.

Customs that had to do with the Christmas tree held the younger children entranced. I could remember Christmas trees from my earlier childhood, before we came to Dakota: the still cold of the winter night, the crunching of snow under our feet as we walked to the church, the roomful of warmth, and the excitement inside. In the front of the church, at one side of the pulpit, would be the tall tree, aglitter with gifts and decorations and the flicker of candles, the latter watched over with some trepidation by our elders.

I had seen all this and remembered it vividly, but most of the younger children in this prairie had no recollection of a really full-grown tree of any kind, and a gaudily decorated one could exist for them only as a fantasy. One morning teacher had varied our Christmas talk by letting each child say what he wished most as a gift, and quite a number of them had chosen a Christmas tree.

Just a few months ago Mrs. Harkness had made a trip back to Pennsylvania to her mother's funeral, taking her little daughter Ann with her. At Ann's first sight of some trees out the train window she had cried out in amazement, "O Mama! Look at the big plants!"

I had heard this story repeated among the grown-ups several times, and it was always greeted with laughter. But it was a homesickish kind of laughter, never very boisterous.

Now when teacher made her looked-for announcement that we would have no more lessons today, and that we should put our school things away, she waited until the crackle of papers, the rattle of slates and slate pencils, and the thud of books being thrust forcibly into desks, had subsided. Then she took a clean eraser and smoothed off every trace of chalk from the middle section of the blackboard. Next, with twenty-three pairs of eyes watching intently, she lifted the lid of her own desk and took out the box of colored chalk.

"Children," she said, "instead of talking about Christmas trees this afternoon, suppose we make one for ourselves, here on the blackboard. Would you like that?"

It was a rhetorical question, answered by an ecstatic chorus of sighing, indrawn breaths. She took up a brown crayon first, and made a few vertical lines in the middle of the lower half of the blackboard.

"We could make the trunk black," she said, "but that wouldn't show so well on the blackboard. So we will use brown. Now how about the rest of the tree? What color shall we make it?"

A half-dozen pairs of small hands waved in the air.

"Green!" several of the children said, but there was a liberal sprinkling of "Purple!" "Red!" "Blue!" choices.

"O, children," teacher said, "didn't we read that Christmas trees are evergreens? So wouldn't green be a better choice for our tree here?"

There was a preponderance of emphatic nods and yeses—but looks of disappointment, notwithstanding, on the faces of the proponents of reds, blues, and purples.

And then, although none of us thought of it as anything unusual at the time, teacher demonstrated that she had the soul of an artist. What matter if trees look green to everyone else? Who knows the color of joy in the eyes of a child?

"It's your tree," she said gently. "We'll make it any color you choose."

Nimbly her fingers manipulated the crayons, using the colors at the children's dictation. First, the network of major branches, then smaller and smaller ones, and finally the twigs. The result was a more pleasing harmony than anyone could imagine, seeing it described dully in print. It was like a green tapestry, with bits of the rainbow glowing through it. Or can it be that it is only a trick of my memory—preserving it thus?

As the tree took shape, the children added further decorations out of their own fancies. The little Lebert girl, a usually shy fifth grader, started it by exclaiming, "That red she is putting on now is a hair ribbon for me!"

Most of the other children took up the game, and teacher let them talk, turning only to give them a brief admonitory look when they became too boisterous.

"I see my Christmas doll!" "My drum is clear on top!" "That's my train, winding 'round and 'round!"

Even my seatmate and I, big girls that we were, could imagine scarfs and handkerchiefs in a maze of colors.

When it was finished, teacher wiped the chalk off her fingers with a dust cloth, and turned to the room with a glowing face.

"So we'll really have a tree of our own this Christmas, won't we?" she said.

One of the Purdy twins raised his hand. "Where will we put it?" he asked.

In an instant the fragile illusion was shattered. There was no longer a gift-laden tree in the room. The thing on the blackboard was only another picture like the ones in books.

It was a few moments before the dismay in teacher's face could be marshaled into something constructive, something with which to meet this crisis. It was a dismay in which impatience or irritation had no part. Only disappointment, modified by pity, that here was one child who had not been able to lose himself with the rest of us in the delights of make-believe.

Meanwhile, like a cloud in the air, there was a question awaiting an answer.

By the time she gave it, teacher's face had regained its composure. With a deliberate slowness that gave emphasis to her words, she told him, "We'll put it right here beside my desk where everyone can see it best."

It was no lightly spoken reply. The hush in the room testified to the solemnity of the moment, as of a vow being spoken, or a name being signed to a momentous paragraph.

The rest of us were completely mystified. Teacher and the Purdy twin were the only ones with any understanding—his on faith, hers on some kind of inner determination that we were unable to fathom.

Then she proceeded to mystify us still further. "We'll have Program Friday this week, too," she said. "Be sure to ask your parents all to come if they can."

Program Friday just before Christmas, when we were only now learning our pieces for the Christmas program? When would we get ready for it? Besides, we had had Program Friday only last week. We usually had it only once a month.

Teacher calmly went on to explain. "We won't learn anything new for this program. We'll use some of the songs and the poems we have had during the year. And don't forget to tell your fathers and mothers we'd like them all to come."

That was some Program Friday! It was the shortest one we had ever had. Just a couple of recitations, and a story the sixth grade had had for a language lesson. Then we all sang "Flow Gently Sweet Afton," and were dismissed.

Teacher told the smaller children they might play quietly for awhile in the back of the room, while she talked to the parents around her desk. We three older ones were assigned to the evening school chores. The boy brought in the coal and kindling for Monday morning's fire, while the other girl and I cleaned the blackboards, dusted erasers, and tidied up in general. Most of the jobs we two did kept us not far from teacher's desk, so we could hear most of what was said.

"I have promised the children a Christmas tree this year," teacher told the group of parents.

Everybody looked amazed, and for a time no one said a word. They all knew, almost to a tree, the only evergreens for miles around. They were the ones on the Carlson and the Evans places. Most of the other settlers had planted some, too, but they had not survived. They all knew, too, the constant tending that had kept these few extant. In the hot summer, during the long July and August drought, when all the wells were low and some of them dry, Sadie Carlson had watered their trees as faithfully as she had their cattle. Pulling up water hand over hand with rope and pail from the stock well near the barn, she had carried it to the thirsting trees every evening after the sun was off them, and was now rewarded by the blessed fact that they were still alive and getting their moisture more easily from winter snows. The Evans trees were a second planting, as their first ones had all died—three rows of little pines, most of them less than three feet tall, set hopefully along the north side of the building lot as a future windbreak.

Cut one of these trees down? It was too unthinkable a suggestion to be put into words, even as a dubious question.

Teacher hastened to explain. "It was this tree I drew for

them on the blackboard that gave me the idea," she said. "I know we couldn't have a pine tree, or any other kind of evergreen. But couldn't we find just an ordinary little tree, or even a bush, somewhere? I thought we could wrap the branches with colored paper. We wouldn't have to use up big pieces; just scraps would do. The children could help me do it, at recess times, so it wouldn't take time from their lessons. I think we could make it real pretty, and they would all love it, I know."

As teacher tumbled out her words with such a pleading urgency to them, the shocked resistance among the group of parents weakened visibly. The director's wife unpursed her mouth, and the tenseness in most of the other faces relaxed.

"Well, I expect we could find some kind of little tree, couldn't we?" one of the women asked.

It was father who put the stamp of finality on the plan. "I've got that bunch of plum brush where Lute's Creek cuts through a corner of my pasture," he said. "We could cut a tree there. Fact is, they could do with a little thinning out."

Other suggestions followed. Quite a few plum trees grew along the Keya Paha River, and most of the settlers knew where there were a few choke cherry trees. Several women shook their heads at this latter suggestion. They needed the choke cherries for jelly ("Even if they don't jell right," one woman interpolated); wild plums were more plentiful.

In the end it was decided to take father's offer, after he reiterated his statement that we could spare a tree from our thicket. It would be most of a day's trip to the nearest point on the Keya Paha, and the road went through numerous draws that were sure to be full of drifted snow. Better to depend on something nearby than to make a long trip at this time of year.

Mrs. Carlson offered a wooden bucket, painted green, that could be filled with sand to hold the tree. She had had geraniums planted in it, but in the first sudden cold snap of the winter she had forgotten to move it back from the window one night, and they had all frozen.

And now to the decorations. Interest had quickened to an excited buzzing of conversation, mostly among the women. There was no one among them who did not have something to contribute. Scraps of colored tissue paper left over from making May baskets or valentines or artificial flowers, ends of fancy shelf paper, carefully hoarded wrappings from a rare box of bon bons, the tinsel lining from packages of tea. One woman had a part of a roll of ceiling paper with silver stars dotted over it. The children could cut them out to make ornaments. Yards of popcorn could be strung, and wound in and out among the branches.

"If we only had some cranberries, like we had back east," one woman said, wistfully. "They make such pretty strings."

"I'd be in favor of eating them, if we had them," her husband countered.

In the fall the McElway girls had strung some of the red seed pods from wild rose bushes. They would be willing to lend them, their mother knew, if they could be put high on the tree out of the reach of the smaller children.

With plans once made, there was no dallying in carrying them out. Before teacher rang her hand-bell for nine o'clock school on Monday morning the tree had been brought in and set in its bucket of sand. It was a drab and scraggly object, in actuality, but we looked at it in the light of what our faith in teacher made of it, a promise of rare joy and beauty.

"When do we fix it?" clamoring voices were asking, as we took our seats. .

But teacher was firm. "We'll practice our Christmas songs for opening exercises," she said, and then to our lessons. Recess is the time for fixing the tree."

Teacher had to relax the strictness of this regime, however, after a few days' try at it. By the time she could get ready the pot of flour paste, and organize the children into cutting and pasting squads, there was not enough time left in a fifteen-minute recess period to do much of the actual decorating.

Recess periods were lengthened to half hours, and there were several longer after-school sessions before the job was finished. Teacher salved her conscience for thus curtailing lesson time by telling us sternly that there would have to be a lot of makeup work done right after Christmas.

But none of us worried about future penalties for today's enjoyment. No schoolroom, no beehive, ever presented a picture of more concentrated industry than our school did in these tree decorating sessions. We older ones did the cutting of the strips of paper, while the smaller children daubed the paste on ends, wiping their sticky fingers with abandon on shirt fronts, overalls, and little aprons. At first teacher gave some concern to the protecting of small garments, but when she saw several of them licking their fingers instead, she decided to ignore the disposition of the surplus paste, restricting her supervision to the mechanics of the decorating job proper.

After the preparation of the strips of paper came the job of applying them to the tree. Teacher and the seventh-grade boy could both reach the very tip of the tree with sufficient ease, so the top flight artistry was allotted to them. Other areas were distributed on down in proportion to the varying heights of the children, and there was work for all. Even the smallest of them became adept at falling in with the work pattern—choose a branch or twig, and a strip of prepared paper estimated to be of the proper length to be wound around and around to cover the twig, with enough lap-over to paste down the end securely.

Teacher countenanced a constant low-voiced chatter as we worked, but she promptly quelled any show of boisterousness as not conducive to efficiency. It was apt to accompany torn strips, spilled paste, and even a tumble of one of the more daring little boys off the edge of teacher's desk, where he had attempted to stand to lengthen his reach.

Occasionally teacher would try to organize the talk with the same Christmas stories and legends we had been having during the school periods. But she found this inadvisable, too, for any prolonged time. She would be working away and at the same time retelling the story of Scrooge and Tiny Tim, or of Bethlehem and the wise men, and look up suddenly to see all hands idle, interest in the story having carried everyone completely away from the job at hand.

Little German Katy, in the primary class, who could speak scarcely a word of English when she started to school in the fall, found all this talk about Christmas, Glory to God in the Highest, and Peace on Earth, too much for her newly sprouting vocabulary to encompass, and she began calling the tree "der glory Baum." When teacher told the rest of us what it meant, a number of the others took up the name in good-natured derision, and in no time at all our tree was universally referred to as the glory tree.

From time to time some of the parents dropped in to see how things were progressing, and from their mysterious, low-voiced conferences with teacher, we gathered they were having some part in our Christmas Eve plans, too. Snatches of conversation I overheard while I was helping the twins with their wraps one evening—in a very dilatory manner, most likely—indicated there had been some discussion of gifts to be put on the tree for all the children alike. Teacher already had a gift for each child, she said.

Someone suggested oranges, but this idea received only fleeting consideration. It was not certain that oranges were obtainable in town, and if they were, who could think of buying twenty-three of them all at once? More than that; there would have to be enough for the small children under school age who would be coming to the program. Oranges were not a staple provision in any of our homes; they were always something special. At our house, for example, an orange was a traditional gift for father to bring home to a sick child who was on the mend and just beginning to have an appetite again.

While this discussion was going on an idea occurred to me, the voicing of which was almost painful to suppress. There stood Mrs. Roberts, not saying a word. Every fall some relatives in Illinois sent the Robertses a barrel of apples from their orchard. And what a pleasure it was to go to the Roberts house in the fall or winter on an errand! Any caller at their house was certain to be treated to an apple before he left, and usually several to take home with him for the rest of his family. Several times Mrs. Roberts had let me go with her to the vegetable cave to get a bowlful of them. Any other cave I had ever been in had the musty, sprouty smell of long-stored potatoes, cabbages, and turnips. In the Robert's cave the only smell was the sweet, tangy one of apples. The apples took over completely. O Mrs. Roberts, I prayed, please give us some apples for the tree!

Mrs. Roberts did not fail me. She was a quiet, dignified woman, and it was her custom to think things out well before speaking. She had married late in life and had no children of her own. She had been a teacher before coming to Dakota, and she still had most of her old school books. My most frequent errand there had been to borrow some of these books to supplement my own texts. I could not understand it then, but when I asked to borrow one of these books after another, she seemed as pleased as though I were doing her a favor. Now, as she offered the apples for the tree she seemed to have the same attitude about them, as though the pleasurable benefits of the gift were accruing to her instead of to us.

From the time the tree project was started I was aware that my mother had some plan of her own about gifts. She did not tell me what it was, at first, but as the time became shorter she needed my help with it in the evenings after the twins and the boys had gone to bed. She was making little baskets of cardboard and stiff paper, and decorating them with fringed tissue paper, tiny paper flowers, and other oddments of color. She made twenty-three of them, one for each pupil and then a larger, very special one, for teacher.

What to put in them called for some discussion. Popcorn was the only treat that was plentiful. Mother longed to make a big batch of fudge, enough to put a piece, or maybe two, in each basket, but Father vetoed this firmly. It would take a week's supply of sugar, and we could not afford that. None of the settlers could afford luxuries of any kind. The payments they were to make on their land within a few months were constantly in their minds, and this opportunity for a deed to land of their own must not be forfeited by careless extravagance. A suggestion that bags of candy might be bought to put on the tree for all the children had been vetoed just as firmly. None of

the settlers felt that they could contribute to such an unnecessary expenditure. So mother contented herself with a compromise filling for her Christmas baskets; each was heaped gener-
ously with popcorn and had a single piece of molasses taffy on
top.

School holidays started the day before Christmas. That
afternoon several of the mothers came to help teacher with the
final arrangements. None of the pupils was allowed to come,
not even the older ones. The last rehearsal of songs, dialogues,
and recitations had been held.

People began arriving at the schoolhouse shortly after seven
that evening. Most of them came in bobsleds, but our family
walked. Having only a half-mile to go, none of us questioned
that it was better for us to walk that short distance, even facing
the icy north wind as we had to do, than to have the horses
standing out in the cold needlessly for several hours. It would be
still colder going home but the wind would be at our backs.

We carried a lantern with us to help us avoid the deeper
drifts, and to keep us from floundering about uselessly in the
snow. A number of the other settlers had lanterns with them,
too, and we used them for light inside the schoolhouse. There
were enough to hang one in each corner of the room and one
behind the tree, and to set one on teacher's desk.

The little room was crowded. Heavy wraps were hung on
the hooks along the rear wall until no more could be accommodated, then laid in piles on the floor, keeping the belongings
of each family segregated, as far as possible, to avoid confusion
in finding them again. People sat on the seats, on the floor, or
stood along the walls. A few had brought their own chairs with
them in the bobsleds. The only clear spot in the room was in
the middle, around the red-hot stove that held sway like a half-
frightening sun, keeping us all comfortable so long as we didn't
get too close. The occasional odor of scorched wool or rubber,
when someone was careless with his coat or overshoes, was a
warning.

But the tree, the fabulous tree, was the center of attention.
Hanging from its multicolored twigs and branches were the
silver stars, the popcorn strings, mother's little baskets, Mrs.
Roberts's apples, and little booklets for all the pupils from
teacher. On it and under it were gifts parents had brought for
their children: dolls, tops, and other toys, and a few gifts for
the adults themselves. These gifts were usually not wrapped,
the name being fastened somewhere on the gift itself, not to a
beribboned box that held the contents a secret. In these gifts,

beauty and sentiment were sometimes sacrificed to practicality. One man bought a washing machine wringer as a Christmas gift for his wife and put it under the tree for her. She said she had needed a new one badly, and appeared well pleased with the thoughtfulness of his selection. Her reaction seemed so genuine one wondered if she might not have scolded him if he had chosen something frivolous for her.

"How could we ever have had a Christmas celebration without a tree?" people asked one another. It was the background for all the performers on the program; looking at it helped to keep the little children quiet; it was the tangible symbol of Christmas joy for everybody.

Tension built up in the room as the program advanced toward the delightful climax of gift distributing. Nothing more was needed, one would have thought, but there was a surprise yet to come. Teacher's mother and father had come over from Gregory County to take her home with them. They arrived late, when the program was nearly over, and had done so with a purpose, it developed. With them was teacher's grandfather who had come in the fall to make his home with his son. He had been a factory worker in Ohio before his retirement, and for years had been in demand at holiday time as Santa Claus for various business firms. He had brought his suit with him when he moved here to his son's home, and he wore it tonight.

It was almost more excitement than the little folks could stand to see the whiskery, red-suited figure, familiar to them in pictures, thus come to life in our midst. Some were too over-awed to move or make a sound; some laughed and clapped hysterically; several of them cried. His arrival and the subsequent distribution of gifts turned the remainder of the evening into a happy hubbub of talking and laughter, crunching of apples and popcorn, mix-ups of gifts and wraps, looking for lost caps and overshoes, a piece of half-chewed taffy caught in one little girl's curly hair.

Before I went to bed that night I set my gifts out on the dresser that I shared with the twins. My booklet from teacher had pansies on the cover and was tied with a lavender silk cord with tassels on the ends. The poem in it was Elizabeth Barrett Browning's "The Swan's Nest." It was in my Fifth Reader. I loved it, and knew it by heart, but this familiarity made the gift all the more pleasing, and the poignancy of the closing lines, "But she would never show him, never, The swan's nest among the reeds," still could bring me close to tears.

There was something I had to think out before I went to

sleep, and it took me a long time. It had to do with my mother and teacher, and Mrs. Roberts. This thinking was prompted by the little baskets mother had made. In some way mother was like these other two women—Mrs. Roberts with her book learning, and teacher with her soft hands and pretty clothes, all of which attributes were so foreign to my mother. Yet in some way she belonged with them; I was certain of it.

After much tortured thinking I was able to define the common denominator of quality possessed by these three as a greater caring-ness for others. Not just her own five children filled my mother's heart. She was concerned for the happiness of them all, in the same way that teacher and Mrs. Roberts were. Yes, these three, among all the women in the community, belonged in a group apart.

This was a wonderful discovery for an adolescent to come upon, and it was my most precious and lasting gift from the glory tree.

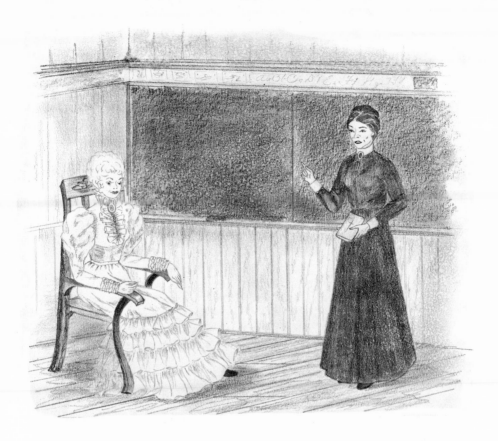

15 / THE PREACHER LADIES

THE SUDDENNESS with which events often happen in childhood must be one of the reasons they are retained so sharply in memory. With no fogging indecisions beforehand, no prodromal warnings, no previously developed and recognized need, they appear like UFO's in the child's consciousness, and indent themselves upon his mind forever.

Such an event was the arrival of Miss Gibbs and Miss Nystrom in the middle of January to hold a series of religious meetings in our schoolhouse; "protracted meetings," as they were called. I know now that these meetings must have been in the planning stage for several months at least. Someone had to have heard about these ladies and their work beforehand. Inquiries must have been made, committees appointed, letters written, arrangements completed, all with the slow goings and comings of the mail since telephone lines had not yet penetrated into the Rosebud Country. I suppose, also, that these ladies must have belonged to some organized religious sect, but I never heard the name of it. Their arrival was my first knowledge of them.

They came by train from somewhere in the East, and father met them at Carlock. Carlock was only eighteen miles away, but it was an all-day trip for father, with Duke and Barney and the bobsled. We had been having frequent snow storms since the middle of November, and there wasn't much left that could be called a road any more. The route was mostly a line of tracks impacted into the snow, going on top of the harder drifts and around the newer soft ones. In several places it even went over the fences. When father drove into our yard he had to get out of the bobsled and shovel a path from the gate to the door, so that his passengers would not get bogged down in the snow when they walked to the house. The boys had shoveled a path early in the afternoon but the snow had continued and drifted it full again.

The preacher ladies, as we called them, stayed at our house throughout the series of meetings. Since building the small addition to the house, we had more room than most of the other settlers. While we were all pleasurably excited at the prospect of having company—even mother, upon whom most of the extra work devolved—the twins and I were not completely happy over it. It meant that we had to give up our bed and sleep in the front room on the floor. This was not the hardship that we had anticipated, however, for mother spread down the old horsehide laprobe with plenty of comforters over it, and except for a mild protest of Marie, "This bed isn't very bouncey, is it?" we found the arrangement very acceptable.

In one respect, it was even a luxury. After the kitchen fire went out this was the only room in the house with any heat in it. It was pleasant to lie there and look at the glow of the fire through the isinglass windows of the hard coal burner a few feet away from us, almost like going to bed without blowing out the light. And for getting up in the morning, it was marvelous. It was the only time we could remember getting dressed in the winter without shivering, except on the occasions of our rare tub baths, which were taken in the zinc washtub in front of the open oven door of the kitchen stove. We learned, however, that our winter baths were not so rare as those of some of the other settlers. The Holland family in our neighborhood were noteworthy in the eyes of the rest of us for their neatness and cleanliness. Yet the father of this family was once heard to exclaim, when the subject of baths was mentioned, "Take a bath in the wintertime? I do that never!")

The ladies held meetings every night in the week, and on Sunday mornings. The boys in the neighborhood took turns going to the schoolhouse early to build the fire, so the room would be warm by the time the meeting started. Father insisted that Floyd take his turn with the other boys, although he was younger than the others, and mother worried about the danger of explosions. On school days there were apt to be a few live coals left in the stove under the ashes from the fire maintained for the school session. Since we had no wood for kindling, the fire had to be started with corncobs and kerosene and the addition of kerosene to smoldering coals is a hazardous procedure. Without saying so, father believed that Floyd was younger than the others only in years, not in capability, so he permitted him to go, after careful instructions about dipping the cobs in kerosene and lighting them before putting them into the firebox.

Entire families attended these meetings. Most of them came in bobsleds, an accepted mode of winter travel. We walked, as we always did to meetings at our own schoolhouse, and the preacher ladies walked with us. Father's ideas of gallantry did not extend to making his horses stand needlessly in the cold to coddle a couple of able-bodied women. Sometimes mother did not go to the meeting. The ladies liked to have a lunch after they returned, and if mother had not had time during the day to fix something, she would stay at home and do it in the evening while the rest of us were gone. There would be doughnuts, or pie, or hot cinnamon rolls, with coffee.

Miss Gibbs did the preaching. She was of a slight, rather angular build, and very trim looking, with her smooth dark hair, her plain white shirtwaists and black skirts, and neatly polished black shoes. She delivered her sermons with a vigorous intensity that left no doubt as to her own convictions regarding her mission in life. Outside the meetings she was reserved to the point of being aloof. She saved herself for our spiritual enlightenment alone. Clearly, hers was the dynamic force that moved these two women from one isolated spot to another on these Dakota prairies, through hardships enough to have provided hair shirts for a whole colony of Christians.

Miss Nystrom was the musician of the team. She played the organ and led in the singing of several hymns at the beginning and close of each service. She was younger than Miss Gibbs, apparently by about ten years. We judged her to be in her early twenties. She was plump, blonde, and full-busted, and her voice poured out into the schoolroom in a soprano flood, making the punier voices of the congregation about as effective as raindrops in Niagara Falls. During the sermon she remained seated beside the organ, facing the audience. She would sometimes smile down at us in a friendly way, and toward the end of the sermon would appear rather fidgety, and leaf through her hymnbook or hold it up to her face to conceal a yawn. She liked all kinds of food, and I used to think she was wondering what we would have for lunch when we got home. She was always jolly and friendly in her associations with us, although proximity to Miss Gibbs never failed to have a restraining influence on her.

One evening after we had eaten lunch I helped mother wash the dishes, then brought my book over to the table where the lamp was, to read for awhile before going to bed. The book was *Martin Chuzzlewit,* and I was almost through it. I looked at the scant number of pages remaining, wondering if it would last until I could get back to the Smiths' house to borrow another one. It was like looking in the cupboard and seeing the likelihood of some unwelcome days of famine ahead.

Miss Nystrom was sitting across the table from me with some crocheting. "Aren't you glad when you get a book finished?" she said to me. "I always am."

That remark set an ocean between Miss Nystrom and me. I was stunned by it, and for a long time I could not thrust it out of my mind. It bothered me to realize how little I knew about how other people think.

I was overawed by the personal belongings of our two guests, and I performed many little services for them with complete willingness because of opportunities thus afforded to look at the things in their room. Their array of blouses—we called them waists—was something to gape at. They had more than I had dreamed any two women could own, requiring all the spare hangers we had in the house. Miss Gibbs's were plain and starchy, but Miss Nystrom's all had lace or ruffles somewhere about them. Miss Nystrom had an enormous set of toilet and manicure articles with celluloid backs and handles, some of which I did not know the names of, or the uses for which they were intended. Miss Gibbs had only a few of these, but they were elegant ones. They all had silver backs, and the mirror and brushes had her initials on them.

It was Miss Gibbs's handkerchiefs, however, that impressed me most of all. I would watch her put away, in the box with the others, the newly ironed ones that I had brought in to her, and was amazed that any one person should own so many. There was never any graceful opportunity afforded me to count them, but I thought there must be as many as thirty. And they were all linen! She told me that most of them had come from relatives in England.

I had one linen handkerchief of my own, a white one, with a sprig of blue forget-me-nots embroidered in one corner. My

Sunday school teacher back in Iowa had given it to me for reading a verse of the Bible every day for six weeks. I treasured it, carrying it only on very special occasions, and then I usually pinned it to the inside of my pocket for safety.

Seeing Miss Gibbs's store of beautiful linen handkerchiefs made me want to show her this one of mine. It seemed to me that it would increase my importance in her eyes, that she would be surprised that I owned such a one, in the same way that she had been surprised to see the Haviland china that Mother used to serve their evening lunches.

I tried to think of some excuse for showing her my handkerchief without seeming obviously boastful, but I could not think of any. So one day I just brought it to her without any introduction to the subject, and said as casually as I could, "I have this one linen handkerchief. Would you care to look at it?"

She told me she thought it was very pretty, but she replied in an abstracted manner, as though thinking of something else, without showing any of the surprise I had hoped for. She left me with the deflated feeling that neither I nor my possessions were very important in her eyes.

If there were any unsavory undertones to the circumstance of these two women living, working, traveling, and sleeping together, I heard no mention of it. So far as I knew, the bond between them was considered to be the Lord's work, and I think they believed it themselves. None of us knew anything about homosexuality; nor, I believe, did either of these two women. It seems to me that each of them found in the other those complementing traits of personality that made her a more complete and satisfied individual, thus obviating the necessity of seeking them in the opposite sex, where they are more commonly found. If their feelings for each other rose to heights of passion, there was always their religion to sublimate them, make them pure and even more ecstatic.

I was able to sense, however, that something about these two women was troubling father. Perhaps it was only the length of their stay. One night after they had been with us about three weeks, I overheard father and mother talking in the kitchen. Father was saying that he thought these meetings had been protracted long enough, and mother was protesting mildly. Mother was never one to have feelings hurt if it could be avoided. I had forgotten all about it by the next morning, but father must have issued an ultimatum some time during the day, for at the close of the service that evening Miss Gibbs announced that the coming Friday night meeting would be their last; they must "accept a call" elsewhere.

On Saturday morning our guests packed their belongings preparatory to leaving, and mother hurried to get some ironing finished for them. She had laid all the handkerchiefs, as she finished them, in one heap on the kitchen table, and asked the ladies to sort out their own. Miss Nystrom selected hers first, and took them into the bedroom to pack them. Then Miss Gibbs sat down at the table and picked them over, one by one, laying her own in a neat little pile ready to put in her box. I sat down to watch her, enjoying one last look at the fragile squares, each with its bit of decoration—hemstitching, embroidery, lace.

Suddenly I barely restrained a gasp, as Miss Gibbs picked up my linen handkerchief and laid it in the pile with her own! I watched her face in an agony of expectation, certain that she would see her mistake. Hers were all white, and mine had those little blue flowers in one corner. But she went on with her sorting, without noticing. She seemed to be thinking of something else, and identifying the linen ones by the feel of them, without really looking at them at all.

As she carried them away, I went into the lean-to that opened off the kitchen, where the boys slept and where the twins usually went to sew their doll clothes. The door was warped, and would not close completely, but I pushed it as far as it would go. I felt very queer, and thought I must look that way, too. I did not want anyone to see me, not even mother. From this seclusion, I listened to the final noises of departure.

The ladies had more to pack than when they came. One woman in the congregation had knitted a sweater for each of them, and others had given them aprons and various other small gifts. They had a difficult time getting their suitcases closed, and finally brought them into the kitchen and asked father to help them.

"Maybe they can't get them closed," I thought to myself. "Maybe they will have to take out some of the things and pack them in a separate box, and then maybe she will notice that one of the handkerchiefs isn't hers."

But with father's help, the suitcases did close. I heard the snap of the locks.

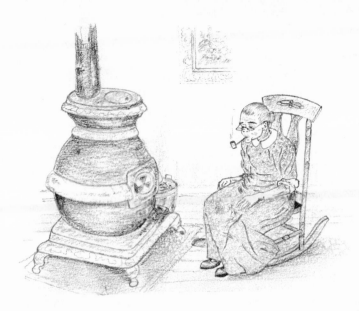

16 | THE TUMOR VICTIMS

THROUGHOUT their stay in Dakota, the Langenfelder family in their sod house continued to exhibit to us a type of culture that we had never known before. Years later, when I started the study of pathology in medical school, I was to recall another novelty they presented me—the first tumors I ever saw to recognize as such. Paradoxically, these were in a husband and wife, cousins of our neighbors, who had come to spend the winter with them. I know now that these must have been benign cysts, his in his lip and hers in an ovary, although the husband referred to his lesion in a proprietary manner as "my cancer" with no trace of alarmed concern.

I have classified these tumors as benign, yet they were visibly invasive and strength-sapping, not to the individuals themselves, but to these relatives upon whom they unloaded themselves for the winter. Were they not malignant, then, to a degree? To which one must reply, "Pathologically, no; sociologically, yes."

We first heard of these Langenfelder relatives on the day before Thanksgiving, when Winnie came over to our house to borrow two cups of sugar. Their men folks would be so disappointed, she said, if they didn't have pumpkin pie for Thanksgiving dinner. The pumpkin had been stewing all forenoon, and Evie had the crusts all rolled out before she discovered there wasn't enough sugar for the filling.

In some respects my mother was a weak character and this was one of her vulnerable spots. As carefully conserved a commodity as sugar was in our household, and in spite of previous experiences with the "borrowing" of these neighbors, she did not have the courage to refuse to contribute to their holiday feast. She could not have enjoyed her own Thanksgiving dinner, she told me later. Mother's conscience was a sentinel that never slept or went off duty. Its monitoring was equally severe in matters of brotherly love as it was with those of devotion to her church and its other Christian principles.

So she measured out the sugar for Winnie, already planning that she could skimp the icing on the cake she planned to make for our Thanksgiving supper, thus insuring that our own sugar supply would not be depleted before we could get to town again. As she handed the bowl of sugar to the grateful Winnie, she noticed that Winnie's eyes were red as though she had been crying. This was most unusual. Battered constantly by hardships as Winnie might appear to anyone else, we never had known her to give way to self pity. She could look cheerful and happy under circumstances that might have driven another woman to think of an overdose of something, or a rope over the rafters. It was the absence of her accustomed carefree look, as much as the redness of her eyes, that was perturbing to Mother.

Sympathy was a commodity that mother never ran out of. Nor did she ever consider events in terms of what a person deserved, or might have brought upon himself. "He hurts," "He is suffering," or "He is unhappy," was all that mother ever needed to know. So now she led Winnie to a chair and sat down beside her, and asked what was the matter.

In a choked voice, Winnie explained. "It's these shoes," she said, pointing to the men's heavy, clumsy work shoes she was wearing. "My own shoes was plumb wore out, and I was supposed to get some new ones when we sold off some of the late hay crop. But then it come time to send the money for Ribb and Eunie's train tickets, and there wasn't enough left to get my shoes."

Winnie sobbed for awhile, as mother murmured words of sympathy, and then she told us the rest of the story. Ribbey was the oldest of the Langenfelder brothers. He and his wife, Eunice, lived in Missouri. During the summer months they were able to get along with what Ribbey made doing odd jobs, such as weeding, hoeing, washing windows, taking care of a neighbor's mules. He explained to his relatives that he couldn't do a steady job, with this cancer and all. His wife having a tumor, too, made them both semi-invalids, so they had to depend on their relatives for their winter support. Winnie did not know how these pathological lesions were incapacitating; she only knew that it seemed the obligation of the Dakota relatives to take care of Ribb and Eunie through the winter, as they had been doing now for three years. Another factor had been making the matter more pressing lately. Granny had been getting more and more impatient to have them come. She liked to get all her family under one roof before the snows started and the roads might be blocked. We had already had several fitful warning November snows. Some of Granny's eagerness, Winnie explained with a faint show of resentment that was unusual for her, was that she looked forward to having someone different in the house, someone new to visit with; Winnie and Evie were just regular family, and they were always so busy. Even though Ribb and Eunie were family, too, they were more like company, with nothing else to do but sit and visit with her.

Ribbey and Eunice arrived a few days after Thanksgiving. Two of the Langenfelder brothers met them in Dallas and brought them and their considerable luggage home in the lumber wagon. I was the first in our family to meet them. When Father went out to do the milking the next morning he saw Old Ike, the Jersey bull, barge through a weak spot in the pasture fence. Deserting his demure harem of Jersey cows, he was now meandering south to see what excitement the mixed herds of Herefords and Holsteins belonging to the Brumbaughs and Fergens might have to offer. I was sent to report his defection to the Langenfelders before he wandered too far away. Old Ike had done this several times before, the last time getting almost to the Nebraska line before his owners caught him.

The smoke from the Langenfelders' chimney always had an acrid smell from the cow chips they used extensively as fuel. The air inside the house was smoky, too, but this was blue tobacco smoke from the pipes of Granny and her four sons. It was a congested family group inside, but cozy and contented and apparently happy. The two new arrivals were seated in the two rocking chairs, and Granny in her favorite low chair beside the stove. The other three brothers were lolling on the beds, Evy was getting the ingredients ready for a stew, and Winnie was washing dishes. When I gave them my message about Old Ike, Barth got up reluctantly from the bed and put on his coat and cap, muttering, "Like to put that ol' son-of-a-gun in a stew!"

Zeke and Luke laughed. "He'd be a tough one to chew," Luke said.

The children and the younger dogs were romping in the available floor space, while the older hounds lay stretched out, dozing, occasionally opening a sleepy eye to watch the shenanigans of pups and children. The youngest two Langenfelders, still infants, had a horse blanket spread on the floor for them, to soften the bumps when they were toppled over in the melee. The faces and arms of these two little ones were flecked by the usual sprinkling of flea bites.

Ribbey was noticeably older than his brothers, and not so stalwart. His hair was beginning to whiten, and there was a pronounced stoop in his shoulders. His so-called cancer was about the size of a hazel nut on his lower lip, near the left corner of his mouth, distorting the shape of his mouth somewhat. The surface of it was smeared liberally with a nauseous looking salve, the color of unfresh egg yolk. This tumor and its landscaping made a horrible focusing point for the eye of the observer, thrusting the other features of his face to the periphery of one's attention. I wondered whether he wiped this salve off before he sat down to the table to eat, and if he did not, how those sitting across from him could retain their appetites; which thought gave me a queasy feeling in my own stomach.

Eunice was an enormous woman—tall, big-boned, and muscular, as well as fat. Sitting in the rocker, her head thrown back and her huge arms resting on its sides, she reminded me of pictures I had seen in my school texts—Michelangelo's Moses, or the biggest Buddha in the world somewhere in Japan. But in Eunice's seated figure there was no indentation for a lap, this angle being filled to the bulging point with the tumor, which looked like a greatly exaggerated pregnancy.

It had been regarded as a pregnancy throughout the early months of its development. It was only after it kept growing on and on without any termination that its true nature was suspected by the patient and her doctor. During the happy months of her expectancy Eunice had made a complete layette, lavishing on it time and money and many dainty stitches. She brought this layette with her when she came to stay with the Dakota relatives, as a lady might carry her chest of jewels. Mother was there one afternoon when she had the garments laid out on her bed for one of her frequent inspections. Were some of the little dresses becoming yellowed? Did some of the tissue wrappings need replacing? A few things needed pressing. It was so difficult to fold them without wrinkling, and perhaps they were packed too tightly in the box. Maybe the next time Winnie heated her irons, she could give them a few touches. Mother thought she could not have been more solicitous if it had been the dreamed-of child lying there on the bed instead of these votive symbols.

In mother's opinion, this layette was indeed a symbol of something to Eunice, a symbol from which she derived pleasure and reassurance. From the time of their first meeting Eunice had strived to convince mother that she and Ribbey were a cut above these down-at-the-heel relatives of his; that they had some appreciation of the finer things of life. The layette was her tangible evidence. It could mesmerize her into a dream world where she could forget her present circumstances—her poverty, her dependence upon people she scorned, her grotesque figure.

In March of that year Evy had another baby, and mother officiated as midwife for the first of several such occasions. It was a job she undertook with reluctance and much trepidation, pressed into it only by the great need. There was too much uncertainty in hoping that the roads would be passable for the doctor from Dallas, eighteen miles away, in the middle of March. It was not much a question of whether he could get there in time, as whether he could get there at all. Besides, there was no money to pay him.

Evy's babies were all pretty little dolls. When mother had this one bathed and ready to dress, she said if she had known where Eunice kept her unused layette she would have helped herself to some of the dainty things to put on this new baby, instead of the coarse, make-shift clothes that were the best poor Evy could provide.

During the last week in March, Ribbey and Eunice began to get restive about going home. They must be there to get their garden in, Ribbey said, and maybe pick up a few odd jobs helping neighbors with their spring work. Eunice concurred with him, but it was plain that her chief urgency was to get away from her cramped winter quarters and her husband's plebeian relatives.

Ribbey's brothers argued that there wouldn't be any gardening possible for a long time yet, as the ground was still covered with snow.

"Not down in Missouri!" Ribbey protested. "It'll be warm and summery there is no time at all!"

The brothers had a very practical reason for imposing some delay in the return trip of their winter boarders. There was the matter of the money for their train tickets; they did not have it. They raised it, finally, by selling two fall calves, at a sacrifice, as they were not in an advantageous marketable condition; but they happened to be desired by a Nebraskan farmer who was building up his herd.

It was a few days after the first of April by the time everything was in readiness, although Eunice had had their bags packed for several days. The three brothers drove them to Dallas in the wagon to take the train. The details of their departure were related to mother afterward by Winnie. At the railroad depot, Zeke gave Ribbey an envelope with enough money in it to pay their fare and to buy groceries for a week after they reached home. Evy had packed a lunch for them to eat on the train.

Ribbey went to the ticket window and transacted his business with a flourish. Then, with an important air, without saying anything to the others, he walked back up the street a half block to a drug store. He returned with some of their best brand of cigars, one each for himself and his three brothers. Mother and I shared Winnie's resentment as she told us the story, but we all laughed about it, too.

"How proud that must have made Eunice!" mother said when she told the story to father that evening.

We all had a mental image of Eunice, wedged tightly in one of the waiting room seats, scarcely large enough to accommodate her, beaming pridefully upon Ribbey as he distributed his treat. Once again her husband had demonstrated his superiority over the rest of his family. Who of them would have thought of the gesture of a parting gift to his hosts? Her Ribbey knew the meaning of noblesse oblige.

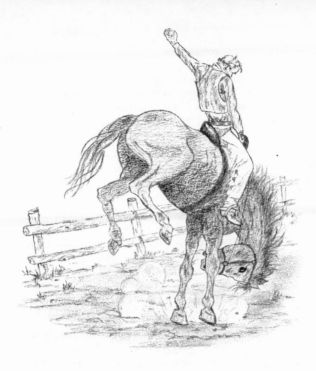

17 | HAZARDS AND SHADOWS

ONE EVENING when the boys and I went to the pasture to drive up the cows, we found that the cover to the stock well had been slipped aside and one of the smallest colts had fallen part way in. He was pawing desperately with his front feet, unable to get a purchase anywhere with his hind feet to boost himself out. He had apparently been struggling for some time, since his coat was darkened with sweat and he looked tired. We were terror stricken lest he fall the rest of the way in and be drowned. It would have been more than the loss of a piece of livestock to us. The colts were all great pets of ours, like members of the family almost. Floyd leaned as far down into the well as he could and grasped one of the colt's hind legs, while Fern and I pulled him as hard as we could by his front feet. With several frantic lunges, through which he might easily have knocked one of us into the well, the frightened and weary little fellow finally got all four feet on earth again and ran off, kicking up his heels in a burst of renewed energy and relief.

We told our parents of the incident, of course, when we returned to the house. Father said nothing, but mother burst into tears, and we heard her telling father afterward, "It might have been one of the children in the well! There are so many dangers in this country; more that we ever knew about before we came!"

131

Poor mother! Nothing to make a shadow, as far as the eye could see, had been her first fearful impression of this new land. She was to learn that the country could make its own shadows on the heart and the mind, if not on the senses. It was not only our unsheltered state, but our aloneness in it, that oppressed her. Firm as she liked to consider her religious faith, there must have been times when not even God seemed very near.

Her concern was mostly for us children. Father was so capable and self-sufficient that she seldom thought of the possibility of danger to him, and she was by nature so completely unselfish as to preclude worry about herself. Her protectiveness could become almost militant, at times, in defense of the boys, who were most in need of it. From our earliest days on the claim, she frequently protested to father, "He is too little to do that!" "They are too young for such work!" "You expect too much of them!" All of which was of little avail. Father would remind her of what he had had to do when a boy—he had earned his own living and helped to support his mother from the time he was thirteen, when his father died. He could not yield to the weakness of sheltering his sons from the rigors he had endured in childhood. They had helped to make a man of him. Were not his sons of as good stock?

So the boys were hard driven throughout their growing years. They would feel rebellious, at times, with fatigue, and with the lack of time for fun and recreation, but they were proud, too, of the adult responsibilities thrust upon them thus prematurely. Seeing the work they were doing in the fields, any observer outside the family invariably thought them to be several years older than they really were.

Mother's fears for them were by no means groundless. Incidents happened that might have had serious or even fatal consequences; it seemed that only luck had saved them. One afternoon Floyd was mowing some wild hay on an unclaimed piece of land about a mile from home. He was driving a team of colts that mother was very uneasy about his taking, but father insisted that they had been working steadily enough to have any troublesome exuberance taken out of them. But they became frightened by a tumbleweed that blew in front of them, and started to run so suddenly that Floyd was thrown off the mower and onto the moving sickle. He caught the horses, quieted them, and brought them back home, not realizing until mother's exclamation of concern called his attention to it, that he had suffered a long, but fortunately shallow, cut on his right thigh from which the blood had soaked through his overalls. The cut healed, however, with no attention other than a cleansing and a firm bandage torn from an old sheet—no tetanus antitoxin, no antiseptic, no stitches.

One accident caused Floyd unforgettable grief, so terrible it did not bear mentioning in the family for years afterward. Father had cut some weeds around a patch of alfalfa. When they were dry he sent Floyd to rake them into piles with the hay rake, whereupon they were lighted and burned. One of the horses hitched to the rake was a skittish mare, and as he drove past one of the burning piles of weeds this mare shied at a sudden leaping of the flames and started to run. She became entangled in the harness and fell into the fire. Floyd worked frantically to loosen the harness and finally got both horses freed, but this one was so badly burned that father rushed to the house for his shotgun as soon as he arrived on the scene and shot her to relieve her of her agony as quickly as possible.

Horses were never dumb animals to us. We reserved that classification to pigs and cattle. Horses could be almost as much company to us as people, and we credited them with intelligence, humor, and a very deep affection for us. We considered Barney the shrewdest of any horse we ever had. To our imaginative minds, he seemed to understand tricks and jokes. On several occasions he untied his own halter rope in the barn by pulling the end of the rope with his teeth. Once we found him untied, and one of the other horses also, and we children always believed that Barney had untied himself and then released his friend, as a double prank, a theory at which both our parents scoffed.

All colts were a delight to us from the time they were born. We could lead any of them without halters, merely by putting an arm around their necks and walking along beside them, and they never kicked at us, even in fun. But they were frolicsome, mischievous little scamps, and the twins were afraid of them. Once one of them chased Marjory around the barn several times, and she, seeing no other means of escape from him, scrambled up the sloping side of a strawstack. To her horror, the colt galloped right up after her! She was almost helpless with fright, and jumped off the strawstack on the other side, whereupon the colt gave up the chase, having seen something else to divert his attention.

We always broke these colts to ride as soon as they were old enough, and we could escape father's surveillance for a sufficient period. His paternal responsibility would never allow him actually to give us permission to ride an unbroken colt, although I suspect he feigned ignorance of our doings in certain instances, knowing what gentle creatures most of these colts were and how accustomed they were to us. We liked to ignore this phase of our adventuring, preferring to think of ourselves as very daring and skillful, riding horses that had never been broken to the -saddle.

Cowboys were our heroes, no other figures seeming quite so dashing or romantic to us. Every festival or carnival worth the name had its bronco-busting contest, in which the cowboys of the neighborhood displayed their skill. There were wild range horses at these rodeos, horses that had almost no contact with human beings, and whose actions were completely unpredictable. They were not circus performers. They meant business, their business being to rid themselves of the encumbrance of man and saddle by any possible means—leaping, buckling their bodies, gyrating, rolling on the ground or running against a fence or building—and loud and long was the razzing the cowboy received who "pulled leather" (grabbed the saddle horn) to keep his seat. Floyd and Fern tried to look and act as much as possible like cowboys. Mother would get very exasperated at them when she saw them trying to walk bow-legged, this being the typical deformity of those who spent much of their growing years in the saddle. Poor Fern was singularly unsuccessful at this, being somewhat knock-kneed to start with.

For several months the boys and I made plans for breaking a pair of rangy gray colts to the saddle. We knew that they offered more of a challenge than anything of the sort we had yet undertaken. They were bigger than any of the other colts we had ridden, and wilder, having spent more of their time in the pasture away from human contact. It was tacitly understood among the three of us that not a whisper of our intentions must reach our parents, as it was certain to be forbidden. Our golden opportunity, or what looked like it, appeared one Sunday. Our parents were invited to have dinner with the Evans family, near Paxton. They left about eleven o'clock, and as they drove out of the yard the boys and I could scarcely restrain our excitement. Mother had cooked some food for us that morning. While I put it on the table for our dinner, the boys would bring the colts from the pasture, and after we had gobbled our meal we could get at the afternoon's fun. We watched the folks drive down the road, but to our amazement and dismay father stopped the team after they had gone only a few yards, gave mother the reins, got out of the spring wagon and walked back to the house. Opening the kitchen door he thrust his head inside and said sternly, "Now I don't want any of you fooling around the gray colts!"

We were dumb with astonishment, unable to imagine what

had made him suspect our intentions. Doubtless we had been poorer dissemblers than we thought.

Not even father's astuteness, however, was able to circumvent all our hazardous and ill-advised activities. One of these happened the week we got a new twenty-two rifle. Mother had not approved the purchase very wholeheartedly, and it was perturbing to her to see how excited and delighted the boys and I were with it, so she saw to it that an immediate restriction was placed on its use. We were never to shoot at anything—targets, rabbits, groundhogs, not even rattlesnakes—unless father was with us. Nothing was said, however, about our taking it out from behind the bedroom door and examining it to see how it worked; so that was what we did on Sunday afternoon when the folks had gone for a ride. We passed it around among the three of us, admiring the smoothness of the stock, the shininess of the barrel, the click the hammer made.

"It's a cinch to load, too," Floyd said, taking a cartridge from the box and popping it into place.

"Then we've got to put the safety on," I said authoritatively, being the oldest. Floyd resisted my bossiness, but I let the hammer back anyway, and in doing so my thumb slipped and the gun discharged. We were a quiet circle of miscreants for a few moments, unharmed, but petrified with fright. We had no hope of concealing the incident from our parents. There was the fresh bullet hole in the middle of the kitchen floor, which seemed to us about as inconspicuous as a chasm from the San Francisco earthquake, still fresh in our minds.

Another occasion upon which father's natural astuteness seemed to have been in abeyance was his purchase of Sadie, a plump, satin-coated bay broncho. He bought her at an auction sale down in Nebraska, at a price that seemed at first like an unheard of bargain. His was the opening bid, a very modest one, and no one bid against him. It developed, however, that he was the only stranger at the sale; the others were all acquainted with Sadie. After father had paid for his purchase, her former owner told him that if no one had bought Sadie he had intended to shoot her, as she was the orneriest, kickingest piece of horseflesh he had ever set eyes on. That very night she proceeded to demonstrate the truth of this appraisal. Father tied her in a stall, and before morning she had kicked out the entire side of the barn within reach of her hoofs. After that she was tied to an isolated post in the barnyard, but, even though unable to hit anything, she still kicked, apparently just to keep in practice. Sadie remained a problem for months, but gradually became civilized, useful, and even likeable. The boys and I insisted that some human being must have been responsible for Sadie's disposition, that she must have been very badly treated when a young colt.

Father's most painful experience with our farm animals was with Yellow Shep, so called to distinguish him from a previous Shep that had been killed by coyotes. Why we did not start from scratch, and give this dog an entirely new name, I do not recall. Yellow Shep was a half-grown pup when we acquired him—in a very casual manner. He followed father home from a sale one day, and we never learned anything about his ownership or his antecedents. We concluded that his previous owner had brought him to the sale with the express purpose of losing him. By the time he was fullgrown he was a larger than average dog of whatever mixture of breed, and completely fearless, as it was easy for him to be, with all the advantage of size and strength on his side. All the dogs in the neighborhood were afraid of him. While father tried to restrain him from any show of viciousness toward other dogs, he did turn Yellow Shep's championship qualities to good account on one occasion. In the Paxton area he passed a farm on his way to town that harbored a mongrel dog with the annoying and dangerous habit of rushing out and barking at every team that passed, following them down the road and harassing the horses for quite a distance. One day father took Yellow Shep with him, ensconced down in the wagon box out of sight. When this mongrel dog rushed out in his usual foray, father took his restraining hand off Yellow Shep's head. With no warning bark, there was a flashing yellow arc over the side of the wagon box, one nip to the annoying dog, and Yellow Shep leaped back into the wagon box beside his master, while the other dog ran yowling back home. Months later, this dog's owner told father that whenever his team came in sight down the road, the dog would run under the porch and hide.

From the beginning, Yellow Shep was strictly father's dog. The dog adored him openly, would follow him anywhere he was permitted, and was completely obedient to him. When he was fullgrown his ecstatic show of affection was sometimes a nuisance to the point of being hazardous. Once when father returned from an all-day absence, Yellow Shep ran to meet him and threw himself against his master with such force that father went rolling on the ground.

From the beginning, Yellow Shep was never as obedient to the rest of us as he was to father, and as time went on, he became increasingly less so. There was nothing lazy about him; he loved to help keep the other farm animals in line, and would do so as assiduously for any of the rest of us as he would for father. Our trouble was in getting him to desist—in calling him off. When a pig got out of the pen, Yellow Shep would keep on chasing it even after it had scrambled back in. When the cattle were being driven to and from the pasture, it was not enough for Yellow Shep to see them walking docilely along the proper paths; he had to nip the heels of the ones in the rear, apparently with a vicious enjoyment.

Father never saw any of this, of course. The dog was a model of rectitude whenever father was around, and intelligently obedient to father's slightest gesture. Mother, however, became more and more worried about the dog, and talked to father repeatedly about him. One of these occasions was after Yellow Shep had turned and snarled at Fern when Fern tried to keep him away from the cats' dish of food.

"I think that dog is part wolf," mother said. "Some day he will kill one of the animals, or maybe even one of the children."

To which father replied, "Oh pshaw!"

Then one day after a business trip to Dallas, father arrived home to find a report awaiting him that he could not ignore. When the boys had driven the cattle up from the pasture that evening, one of the smaller calves had gamboled about behind the rest of the herd for a little extra activity before retiring for the night. It became frightened when Yellow Shep attempted to drive it up to the body of the herd, and panicked, running about wildly in every direction, with the dog now at its heels, now at its head, as excited as the calf was, with deadly intent, tearing at the calf's heels, throat, and flanks and leaving numerous strips of hide torn and bleeding. Both boys had been terrified.

"I sure thought he was going to kill that calf," Floyd said, and Fern added, "When we started to try to pull him away from the calf, he turned around and grabbed one leg of my overalls in his teeth."

Father said little, but it was clear to him that there was some action to be taken, and that it was his duty to take it. There was no one else at hand for such a job. We did not even know the name of any veterinarian. The next morning when the boys had gone to the field and mother and I were in the yard feeding the chickens, we saw father walking out toward the pasture with his shotgun over one arm, and Yellow Shep bounding along beside him. We went back in the house and shut the door, but we heard the shot, anyway, and a few minutes later father brought his gun in and put it away, and went out to the tool shed for the spade.

18 / THE BONE MAN

ONE JULY MORNING a tent appeared at the foot of a butte about a mile and a half south of us. The twins saw it first, when they went to the far pond with Rover to help him chase frogs into the water, a favorite sport of all three of them. They were back at the house by noon, when father came in from the field for dinner, and they told us about it, excitedly.

The prospect of more new neighbors was always an interesting and pleasurable one, but father's reactions in this case were mixed. "That means we won't get any more wild hay off that piece," he said. "I was fixing to cut that slough again this fall." Then he added, puzzled, "It beats me how anybody could think there's enough good farm land there to make it worth breaking up. It's mostly rock and sand."

We could see a figure moving about the tent at intervals, but we could not determine what he was doing. He had no lumber with which to be building. He hadn't even a horse, and a man alone on the prairie without even a horse is an impotent being, indeed. How could he and his tent have arrived there, we wondered.

Our questions were answered about the middle of the afternoon, when Roy Brumbaugh drove by to give us the news. The stranger was having his meals with the Brumbaughs, and it was Roy who had brought him and his equipment to the spot where he was working, and helped him to set up his tent. He had come up from Nebraska, not from the railway station at Dallas, which was the reason he had not passed our house. His name was Dr. Troxell, a book kind of doctor that didn't have anything to do with sick folks, Roy said. He was a school-teaching fellow from a place called Ann Arbor, and he had come here to spend the summer digging up the bones of old dragons. Roy made this last statement half sheepishly and half defiantly, as though he expected to be laughed at for his gullibility.

The boys and I were wild with excitement.

"A stranger from away off in Michigan finding something in our prairies worth spending his summer to dig out!" I marveled. "And something we never suspected was there!"

Floyd told the twins that maybe some of that howling we heard at night was really dragons instead of coyotes, and had them both crying in terror until mother made him stop his tormenting.

The next morning father caught Fern dragging his best post-hole spade down to the creek with him. He thought it might be softer there· to dig, Fern explained, and maybe he could find a dragon all his own and sell it for enough money to

138

buy a bicycle like the ones in Montgomery Ward's catalogue, the mail-order catalogue being a constant among all the settlers. The price of any contemplated purchase was looked up in "the catalogue"; women went window shopping in "the catalogue"; children's letters to Santa Claus were inspired by pictures in "the catalogue"; when women did their sewing they looked in "the catalogue" for ideas about styles. The most common reply to such a question as, "My, where did you get that pretty new dress?" was, "Oh, I sent for it." After the rural route was established, people put up large-sized mail boxes to accommodate mail-order packages.

Father never ordered anything from a mail-order house with a perfectly clear conscience, however. He remembered his store-keeping days in Iowa, and his deadly enmity toward such houses as Sears Roebuck and Montgomery Ward, and he never got over being a little ashamed of anything we had from them. For people as remote from merchandising centers as we were, however, ordering things by mail was the only way to have any choice of selection, sometimes the only way to get them at all. Also, it was usually the most economical way, arguments to the contrary notwithstanding. Merchants argued that you got what you paid for, that cheaper goods were inferior, but the settlers said, philosophically, that they "would do."

Years later, at the University, I heard a youth remark that he had often heard his parents recall with pleasure the good old days when they were very young and had very little in the way of worldly goods, when they would spend long winter evenings sitting by the fire with a catalogue, looking at the pictures and wishing for things. Once when my husband and I spent an evening at the Hall home, Lorene brought out a Sears Roebuck catalogue for the year nineteen hundred, which she had found when sorting over some of her mother's things in the attic. The four of us found much interest and entertainment in looking through it, the pictures furnishing an entire panorama of the living of that era. (This was years before an enterprising publisher brought out one of these old catalogues in book form.)

This catalogue-inspired daydream of Fern's came to naught, however, as many of Fern's daydreams did. Father ordered him to put the sharp, gleaming, rust-free spade back in the tool shed, and Fern had to content himself with an observer's interest in the excavating project, without participating.

The news of the strange doings on this prairie hillside soon spread, as news does, even across prairie distances, and Dr. Troxell began having daily visitors, to all of whom he was very affable, and willing to explain his peculiar work. He was a paleontologist from the University of Michigan, who had been working earlier in the summer in northern Nebraska. While there he had heard a rumor, later verified, that a settler in the southern part of our county in South Dakota had come across some peculiar bones, while digging post holes. The discovery had so roused this farmer's curiosity that he had spent the rest of the morning in scientific ardor, digging out the bones with a spade. This circumstance was a grievous one to Dr. Troxell, glad as he was to get the bones at all, for when he examined them he discovered a number of the prize specimens damaged badly by the crude and vigorous manner of their excavation.

Dr. Troxell's digging site was within easy walking distance from our house, and we often went down to watch him work. It looked like a slow, tedious job, more painstaking than most jobs we had ever seen done. It seemed more nearly in the category of baking a fine cake or making a neat page of letter-writing than in working with farm soil. He used a small chisel to dig away bits of earth until he came to the surface of a specimen, then he brushed off the last dust from the bone with a soft paint brush. Most of the large bones were already cracked across in several places, and had to be removed in pieces. As they were removed, they were placed on a slab carefully, in the proper juxtaposition, and coated immediately with shellac to prevent further disintegration from contact with the air.

Dr. Troxell was quite jubilant over his finds, prizing particularly a jawbone which measured about five feet. From the measurements of the bones he found, he constructed for us the dimensions of the whole mastodon, life-sized, a monster such as most of us had never dreamed had really existed. There were some who doubted it anyway, refusing to believe the evidence of their own eyes' perceiving. Dragons were no more incredible. To me, all this made the face of the prairie more Sphinx-like than ever, and I wondered vaguely, half fearfully, what other secrets possibly were hidden beneath her rippling inscrutability.

A lone, isolated little store building called Eastview was located about two miles beyond the place where Dr. Troxell was working. Its owner had dreamed of a bustling prairie city at this site, but his dreams had failed to materialize. He had planted a grove beside his store building, and once when he had been away on a trip he wrote a letter to the Gregory County paper saying how wonderful it was to get back to "the beautiful hills and green trees of Eastview." The trees all died the first year, no other building had ever been erected in Eastview, and this store building had now been empty for some months. This saga of failure and despair made a fortunate circumstance for Dr. Troxell, however. This empty building afforded him a place to store his specimens, the only building for miles around that was available for such a purpose. Every evening he would take his day's find, all carefully shellacked, to this building to be housed until his excavations should be completed. He even bought a new padlock for the door, and never failed to lock it after him, to everyone's amusement. Nobody ever locked things up in this country! And who would steal stuff like that, of all things?

Dr. Troxell gave two lectures during his stay among us. The first was at Springview, Nebraska, where he had previously found some other specimens. He asked Floyd to drive him down there. We had our first car by that time, a Buick touring car. Father was away at the time, and mother was rather loath to give her consent, but Floyd won her over, as he could usually do. Father was not pleased when he learned of the project. It was a long, rough, stony road to Springview, made for wagons or saddle horses, rather than cars, and very hard on tires. My friend Hazel, later my sister-in-law, and I went with them. I have wondered since, knowing more about such things than I did then, whether Dr. Troxell had planned to think over his speech en route. It was just as well if he had not, for he had little time to concentrate on it, with such a chattering group with him. His speech, however, interesting and intriguing as it was to us, was probably only his most elementary classroom talk, as his hearers were ill prepared to assimilate more than that.

We reached Springview in the late afternoon, and drove around for awhile and looked at the town. We had supper at a little frontier restaurant—Dr. Troxell called it "dining"—where everyone sat down together at a long table. The table was full when we arrived—a number of cowboys, farmhands, and cattlemen appeared to be remaining in town for the evening, and I saw some of them later, at the lecture—so we sat back in some weather-beaten but comfortable old rockers to wait until they had finished eating. When a sufficient number of places were empty, the waitress plunked down some heavy plates and started to toss out the silver. Then she glanced dubiously at Dr. Troxell. His eastern look and well-cut clothes had their effect. With a half-embarrassed uncertainty she picked up the plates and silver again, went to the sideboard and got a handful of paper napkins from a tall glass, which she spread over the spots on the tablecloth left by the first crew. Then she set our places.

After supper we went to the home of the woman who had made the arrangements for the lecture. The three of us—Floyd, Hazel, and I—were strangers in the town, and we accompanied the celebrity, which gave us a feeling of importance. The celebrity was very considerate and did nothing to deflate this feeling. He took care to introduce us to all who came up to talk to him, both at the house and at the town hall where the lecture was held. After his talk an informal reception gave anyone desiring it an opportunity to meet the honored guest and to ask questions. The reception was brief, for although a great many people stayed, not many of them had the courage or the background of information to ask questions, and their contacts consisted mainly of awed handshakings.

By popular request, Dr. Troxell repeated this lecture a short time later, for the benefit of the people in our neighborhood, and it was a lecture unique both to lecturer and to audience. It was delivered under what were probably the strangest circumstances in Dr. Troxell's lecturing experience, and it was probably the strangest tale the group had ever heard. It was held on a pleasant Sunday afternoon, in Custer's pasture; in the open air, with no platform, no seating arrangements—only the gleaming sunlight, the rippling breeze, and the grassy hillside. No building in the vicinity could have accommodated the crowd.

The audience assembled in a semicircle, some seated in their vehicles, some on the grass. And here, where the monsters themselves once roamed, a punier race heard the story of their age, told over their helpless bones thousands of years after. Reading one group of Edna St. Vincent Millay's sonnets, "Epitaph for the Race of Man" brings this scene vividly to my mind.

Listening to the man's talk, the faces of these settlers displayed a variety of emotions—awe, wonder, intense interest, bewilderment, skepticism. To us, the Revolutionary War seemed a long time ago, and here was one who spoke of time in terms of a million years! The pious ones among his hearers were disturbed because they could not conciliate what he said with statements in their well-worn Bibles. Yet there were the bones themselves, beside him as he talked, as irrefutable evidence! Many of us were confused for a long time afterward by what he told us.

Dr. Troxell's summer with us was an important event in our lives, one that we discussed a great deal. We always referred to him as "the bone man." Our psychology was such that we were interested in everything, especially the new and unusual, which gave us a sense of growing and developing along with the country. There was none of the feeling that the status quo was already established, as in the older places we had come from; things finished, all laid out in section lines like our roads; customs and conventions already ossified. Difficult as it was to work things out by ourselves, it was much more zestful. I have always felt in harmony with this aspect of pioneering. To me, certainties become boresome. I prefer the hoped-for perhapses, even though so many of them never materialize. It is the appetite that matters; the pleasure fades with satiation. Again, with Miss Millay, "Let me lie down lean, With my thirst and my hunger."

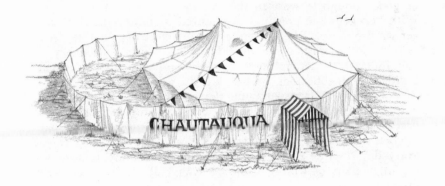

19 / CHAUTAUQUA

THE *Gregory County News* was published once a week. One announcement it carried early in every summer, read by all subscribers with intense interest and anticipation, was that of the annual chautauqua. Nearly everyone aspired to one or two offerings, at least, of this glorious entertainment. A season ticket afforded the height of the year's theatrical pleasure. One summer, in the same mail that brought the paper containing the announcement, came a letter for me from my good friend Katherine, inviting me to spend the entire five days of chautauqua at her home in Dallas. I could hardly bear the suspense until it was finally decided I might go. My going was dependent upon a number of considerations; whether mother could spare me, whether father could afford the time to take me there and bring me back again, whether we could afford the money that would be required for my season ticket, and whether I had clothes enough to carry me through five whole days of dressing up and going places every afternoon and evening.

All these requisites were finally declared feasible, and I wrote her my acceptance, after which mother and I started getting my things ready. I had one white dress which Aunt Susie had made for me the summer before; quite an elaborate dress, with many tiny tucks, and rows of lace and insertion. It was one of the laws of propriety with Aunt Susie that any young girl ought to own one good white dress. I had a light tan voile dress also and a middy suit of white linen that was considered wearable to away-from-home functions when all available supplies were needed. My least-worn, everyday dress of calico would be good enough to wear in the forenoons at Katherine's house. With between-time pressings, we figured I could make this meager wardrobe do. The tan voile was my most dependable dress, as it could be washed out quickly by hand, when necessary. I had four white petticoats, with tucks and ruffles of wide embroidery at the bottom. A girl had to wear two of these at a time with a thin dress—having the outline of her figure show when standing in the sunlight was a disgraceful and humiliating occurrence, always to be guarded against. I owned only one pair of good shoes, and they were white and would need to be cleaned every day, mother cautioned me. These, with my underwear, my three pairs of white cotton stockings, all my handkerchiefs, my purse, and my Japanese fan, constituted my chautauqua-going equipment. I longed for a white parasol like Katherine's new one, but I knew I could not have that. Katherine was an only child, and it was to be expected that she could have more things than I, the oldest of five.

I had become acquainted with Katherine the first year I attended high school in Dallas, and her friendship meant a great deal to me, being the first intimate, lasting one I ever had with a girl of my own age. The friendship had been mostly of her seeking, however; I should never have thought of making overtures to her. She was entirely different from me, having many qualities which I lacked, but which I admired intensely. She was very pretty—beautiful, in fact—small-boned and slender, with dark curly hair and Irish blue eyes and complexion.

Katherine had two failings that were a source of some disturbance to her parents. She could not carry a tune, and she could never learn to spell. She was an honor student, always, except for her spelling. Throughout her grade school years her parents had struggled to bring her spelling up to her other scholastic attainments but to little avail. By the time she was through high school they were almost resigned to her using her own unique methods of putting letters together to make words. Early in her college career she corresponded with a boy friend from high school days. After the exchange of the first few letters he suggested to her—very delicately, he probably thought—that for their mutual improvement they could criticize each other's composition and spelling. A choice recollection of mine is a letter I had from her once, telling me of a friend who was ill with "jondiss." Katherine's spelling was logical—that much could be said for it. There was seldom any doubt in the reader's mind what word she meant.

I was at Katherine's home a great deal during my high school years, and the hospitality was a valued part of my social education. I was often invited to their house for meals, which were enjoyable in every way. They never fussed through an entire orthodox dinner menu, as we did at home, but fixed one or two things that best suited the fancy of the moment, and garnished the whole meal with entertaining and edifying conversation.

Katherine's mother was one of the most interesting women I ever knew. She had been a beauty in her youth, too, and was still handsome, but prematurely aged in appearance, mostly because her hair had become snow white. Age had slowed her physical activity, also, but not her wit. Her gift of humor was a constant delight, and sparkled her conversation, so that if she were talking in a room, one instinctively wanted to draw near enough to hear. She was a good story-teller, and I loved her anecdotes, having many private chuckles over them afterward, all to myself. She told once about having had to be taken out of a minstrel show in Denver, because she laughed so hard she became hysterical. Another story was about the first cake she made after she was married. Both she and her husband were so surprised and delighted over its perfection that they sat down on opposite sides of it, each with a fork, and ate until they met in the middle. She had been a teacher in Ouray, Colorado, in her early years, and once tutored Mrs. Evalyn Walsh McLean.

Katherine's father was a much more quiet, stable person, but he had his own brand of wit. He coined what I believe to be the most elaborate epithet I ever heard. When he became exasperated at his daughter, Katherine, for some impish piece of childishness, he would say to her, "Why you great big stand-up-in-the-corner-and-bawl-for-buttermilk-when-you-know-there's-not-a-drop-in-the-house!"

Father and I were up early for the long drive to Dallas on the morning of the hot July day that chautauqua opened. We drove past the school grounds on the way to Katherine's house. The tent was already up, and the men were arranging the last of the plank seats. Katherine and I would be attending every performance. The afternoons were blistering hot, but we would not have dreamed of staying away on account of the heat, or for any other reason we could think of. We had season tickets, and to miss a performance would be throwing away that much entertainment. Occasionally one would hear some blasé adult say that he or she did not go to a certain performance—it was too hot, or too tiresome to go all the time. I never could believe that this was anything but an affectation.

Chautauqua week was always a part holiday for everyone. Only the most necessary tasks and services were kept going.

Housewives did only a sketchy amount of cooking during that five days, asking their families to subsist on a sort of picnic standby consisting, so far as possible, of foods that could be prepared beforehand—pastries, baked ham, or meat loaf that could be eaten in cold slices, a big pot of baked beans. The occasion itself imposed extra tasks on the housewives—the pressing of light, easily crushable dresses, the washing of hose, the cleaning of white shoes—all necessary to keep presentable under the strain of so much going. All this, with attending two performances a day, and getting the children off to practice for the pageant in the mornings, made a hectic week.

I venture to surmise that nowhere in their circuit did the entertainers receive heartier applause and a more personal welcome than they did in Dallas. Plays, readings, musical numbers were encored again and again. If there is any substance to the stimulus that entertainers are supposed to receive from the enthusiasm of their audience, then these entertainers, and the lecturers as well, must have given us the best they had.

Chautauqua was indeed a boon to people like us, starved for entertainment. I have thought since that a part of the pleasure we derived from the lectures was because we never anywhere else heard such a fine easy flow of correctly spoken English. It was a form of music to me. I remember thinking that one lecture in particular was the finest, wittiest, most polished address I had ever heard, and probably it was. One group of players was encored so persistently and with so much enthusiasm that they used every scrap of their repertoire, collective and individual, and finally closed with a skit that was patently mostly impromptu, and they seemed to enjoy it as much as the audience did.

Sometimes, walking past the dressing tents, we caught exciting glimpses of some of the performers themselves. They were real theatrical folk to us, beings from another world. Frequently these entertainers were invited to meals in the homes of Dallas residents. I used to wonder what it would be like to sit down at the same table with one of these glamorous beings. Not that I ever really wanted to; it would have been painful to me. I knew I should have been tongue-tied and paralyzed with shyness.

It would have been difficult for me to choose which type of program I enjoyed most. I was enthralled by the lectures, but in the plays and the musical and reading numbers there was the added delight of all the lovely clothes. Whatever the number to be presented, when the director had finished his introductory speech and the tent flap on the left or right was pushed back to admit the personnel of the program's offering, I felt that thrill of anticipation comparable only to the opening of the most interesting looking package on Christmas morning.

Thomas H. Duncan's novel, *O Chautauqua,* describes the same chautauqua I knew, also, notwithstanding the insistence of many good people to the contrary. The atmosphere is all there in his book, but his is the satirist's tongue-in-cheek appraisal. I did not see it like that. I was the enraptured country girl, seventh row from the front.

20 / ACCESSORY PIONEERS

MILTON I. ELLIS, the father of my friend Katherine, was a Dakota pioneer who never rode a horse or followed a breaking plow. He was one of the considerable group upon whom the workers of the soil depended for some refinements of living for themselves and their families beyond the realm of the merely physical. Among these were the occasional doctor and dentist, the businessmen with their varieties of goods and services, the preachers and teachers. In this group, Mr. Ellis remains outstanding in my mind, being one of the finest teachers I have ever known.

Looking back upon that time, it seems to me that Mr. Ellis must have felt fully as great a spirit of adventure as any of the homesteaders, coming as he did to be superintendent of schools in this new town in a new country and a new schoolhouse. He had little supervision, few restrictions except those imposed by the stringencies of material resources, and his blueprints for teaching were mostly those in his own head, of his own devising. He had freedom to use his talents as he felt inspired to do, which, in a gifted person, is the most propitious setting for the production of good work.

I think of him, and his comparatively untrammeled teaching job, when I hear our contemporary teachers talk about their work. "I love teaching, but——," such a conversation is apt to begin, followed by harassing details that make teaching sound like something other than a halcyon occupation—jungles of paper work, increasing strictures from the hierarchy above, tightened regulations within the system, rules beyond reason.

"My principal refuses to accept the fact that there are subnormal mentalities," a special education teacher told me. "If a pupil doesn't function up to the average level, the only explanation that he will consider is that the teacher isn't doing her job. He must fit everybody into his guidebook rules."

Another teacher made some scathing remarks about two courses she was required to take to qualify for a degree and an increase in salary. Neither was a course she would ever be expected to teach since in her school system they were covered in special departments. "These subjects will not broaden my education in any way, or make me a better teacher," she said. "I figure that by taking them I am just buying a degree."

Mr. Ellis, in his work, faced a sufficient number of challenges to make him dredge up all the skill and ingenuity he could muster in addition to his academic qualifications which were considerable. Dallas was immensely proud of its new schoolhouse. We were convinced it was the latest design in educational facilities. Accustomed as I was to our cramped living quarters in our claim shack, the stairs in the new school were a symbol to me of progress and of expanded opportunities. Walking up those stairs daily gave me the feeling that I was going somewhere, in the fullest, most important sense. It never occurred to me that Mr. Ellis could be seeing, as he doubtless was, all the things our fine new building lacked, and that one of the challenges he faced was devising ways to compensate for its shortcomings.

Our new school building had no gymnasium, for one thing, an unthinkable omission by present standards. (In the minds of some planners the gymnasium would be the focus of consideration, with the rest of the school built around it.) Mr. Ellis was not one to see athletics neglected in his school, however. He organized a track schedule, and a football team, also a girls' basketball team which he coached himself. Having no inside court, we played in the open air beside the schoolhouse. Our games were thus subject to the permissibility of the weather, and the support of our fans was hampered by the fact that there were no seats for spectators.

Another lack, unthinkable by present standards, was laboratory space. Our science courses, including Mr. Ellis's physics class, were purely classroom affairs, conducted with the aid of a textbook and whatever accessory enlightenment could be provided by the ingenuity and erudition of the instructor. Mr. Ellis's accomplishment that perhaps approximated most nearly pulling a rabbit out of a hat, was his organization of a class for the high school girls that had to take off without either laboratory or textbook or even a course of study. This was his embryo home economics department, conceived in his mind and born into a cooking class, taught by a series of the town's best cooks, who lectured and demonstrated to us, in turn, in their own kitchens. These classes were held once a week, immediately after the regular school session was finished at four o'clock. Some of these provisional teachers told us things that have remained indelibly in my mind. One of these was by the woman who gave us the lesson on pastry. "Be very cautious about the amount of water you use," she told us. "Add it as though every drop cost a dollar." The value of the dollar in those days made this a striking analogy.

Within the week after each of these lessons, each student was required to concoct in her kitchen at home an example of the week's subject, to be graded by her mother. As these grades came to Mr. Ellis's office, an inevitable weakness of the system became glaringly apparent, causing him to tell us, with the twinkle in his eye that always took the sharp edge off his sarcasm, to inform our mothers that 100 percent was absolutely the highest grade that could be recognized, and that averages even approaching that mark would have to be regarded with skepticism.

Mr. Ellis's manner of expressing amusement was one of his most engaging characteristics. It seldom burgeoned into outright laughter, but flickered across his face from the crinkles at the outer corners of his eyes to the tiny ripples that encased his smile, and erupted finally into a quiet chuckle. The effect was to make us feel not laughed at, but participators in a humorous situation. In some indescribable manner, he was able to express at the same time, the underlying seriousness in what he was saying to us. It is thus that I see him most vividly in memory; a neat, stocky figure in a gray suit, standing before us in the assembly room in a purposeful stance, having in mind a carefully thought out communication he must relate to us for our betterment. His head, more than any other I have ever known, is most aptly described as leonine, rising as it did from a forceful breadth of shoulders, and topped with a thick mane of wavy, graying hair, usually in some disarray, as though tossed about by vigorous physical activity, or rumpled by running his fingers through it in tortured thought.

One such speech he made to us was a partial retrenchment from a position he had taken previously, and his amusement, in this instance, was directed inwardly toward himself. It was a speech mainly to the athletes. He said that recent events on the football field had led him to believe that in some of his previous talks about fair play, and knowing how to be good losers, his rhetoric had apparently obfuscated some equally valid considerations; namely, that winning is one of the objects of a game, and that beating a competitor fairly is in no wise reprehensible.

A concomitant circumstance of Mr. Ellis's teaching career in Dallas that must have given him no dissatisfaction was his supporting personnel in the high school. They seemed to me, and still do, in retrospect, to be people of the highest caliber, personally, as well as being excellent teachers. There was Walter Frankenfield, "Frankie," a bright, attractive young man who came to Dallas for several years and then spent the rest of his life at the State University, first as a student and then as a faculty member.

The two I knew best were Elizabeth Bisbee and Theresa, "Tec" Coffman. It would be difficult for me to recount the various kinds of education I had from these two young women. Much of it was intangible, fruit of my first acquaintance with just-out-of-college personalities, with their mixture of sophistication, exuberance, confidence, ambition, and dedication to the job at hand. They were graduates of the Iowa State Teachers' College, at Cedar Falls (now the University of Northern Iowa), and it was from them that I first heard of this institution. With alumnae like these to boost the school by praise, precept, and example, it is easy for me to understand how it has attained its high rank in our educational system. Between them, these two taught me English, German, Latin, mathematics, and many other things. Their interest in students was not bounded by the subject matter in the courses they taught. It embraced all the attributes of a student's character and personality. I think I was a challenge to them in these extracurricular respects, being a shy, awkward, uncouth country girl, badly in need of tutoring in social graces, attention to personal appearance, carriage, and manners.

It was necessary for me to live in Dallas while attending school there. The first year I worked for my board and lodging, with a family named O'Neill. Mrs. O'Neill was a blonde, energetic little woman of German descent. She had social aspirations, and was an excellent cook and housekeeper. I might have learned a great deal from her if I had been more interested and less homesick so much of the time. Her husband was a traveling salesman. My contribution to their household economy must have been of dubious value, consisting of little more than the evening dishes, baby-sitting for the little boy, Jack, and helping with cleaning on Saturday.

The next year Edith Smith and I had an attic apartment in which we did light housekeeping. This was a good arrangement, and for the most part I was happy and contented. I continued to have bouts of desperate homesickness, however, which caused me acute mental suffering. I was able to get home about once a month; at longer intervals during the depth of the winter when there was always the uncertainty about being able to get me back on Sunday evening. Getting me home meant a lot of driving for father or the boys at best; and it was not to be expected at all if a blizzard or a spell of bitter cold was likely.

I always hoped they would be coming for me, no matter how bad the weather was. When they were not waiting for me when school was out on Friday afternoon, I would go downtown about noon on Saturday and walk up and down the street, looking in the stores where they usually traded, hoping so much that some of them would be in town, yet telling myself that if they didn't come on this Saturday they would be all the more apt to come on the next. I think I endured longer intervals of absence better than the shorter ones, and probably would have suffered less if I had been so far away that there would not have been this tantalizing hope recurring every weekend. As it was, I could not rid myself of it, try as I did to distract my mind in other directions. The homesickness befogged every other thought, every other desire. So I walked up and down, looking first at the teams tied to hitching posts along main street—looking for the sorrels, Nell and Gypsy, if they had come with the spring wagon, or Duke and Barney with the lumber wagon. (We did not have our first car until after I had finished high school, and was away at the University.)

In the season of snows, which was most of the winter and sometimes into the spring, the conveyance I would be expecting —hoping—to see was Duke and Barney hitched to the bobsled. I sighted them with joy, knowing full well what the trip home would be like. I would be wearing my warmest clothing—long underwear, of course, and heavy stockings; petticoat, a woolen school dress, my heavy winter coat, woolen hood, scarf, mittens, and overshoes. There would be a layer of straw in the bottom of the bobsled, in which we sat, with a horsehide robe over us, and several rocks at our feet, which father had had reheated at the livery stable or some other obliging business place, just before we started. All of this was feebly insufficient protection from the cold and the biting wind. At the beginning, our faces suffered most. We would try shielding them with our arms, snuggling lower into our coat collars, readjusting scarfs over our faces, turning our heads against the wind, which father could do even while driving, as Duke and Barney could be trusted to pick their route. Scarfs must not cover our faces completely; our frozen breaths would soon impregnate a scarf with an uncomfortable icy patch. So our breath, like that of the horses, escaped into the air in a visible, icy vapor.

As we drove along, however, certainly by the end of the second hour, our feet would be the part of us that suffered most from the cold. We would move our legs about, readjust the robe, wriggle our stiff and aching toes as best we could inside our heavy foot coverings. Nothing helped very much. Our feet grew colder and colder, and were so painful that I had to exert myself to restrain my tears, which would soon have been drops of ice on my cheeks. Then father would get out and walk beside the bobsled, and insist that I do so, too, although I was in such misery that I could scarcely exert myself to that extent. Walking was the proper procedure, a preventive therapy. It stimulated the circulation in the painful extremities. The pain was still there, but preferable to the relieving numbness, which would mean that the feet were literally frozen.

I never asked myself whether getting home was worth all

this. It would have been a rhetorical question. Nor did I ask myself whether father thought it worth all this physical effort and discomfort. I took that for granted, too. Our family was not demonstrative in the usual ways, and we were better at deeds than words or gestures. Mother would have cooked her welcome, and the kitchen was redolent with her art. Fresh baked bread and cinnamon rolls mingled their aroma with that of roast beef or pork and their vegetable accompaniments—among them probably a hubbard squash brought up from the cave, its green shell as hard as when picked in the fall, chopped with a hatchet into irregular segments resembling pieces of broken crockery, and baked in the oven beside the roast. By the time a piece was served on a plate it would still be so hot that the gob of butter put on it would slide off immediately and have to be scooped back up and mashed into the mealy yellow layer. We all ate prodigiously, stopped just short of total possible intake by the mute reproach of the mince pies on the ledge of the kitchen cabinet, "Leave room for us."

Conversation, sketchy during supper, burgeoned immediately afterward into a constant flow while mother and I were doing dishes, and continued throughout our waking moments until it was time for me to leave again after Sunday dinner at noon. I gorged hungrily all the trivia of home—the doings of the neighbors, the new kittens, the smart tricks of the dog, the welfare of the horses, mother's quilt-making project, the twins' grades at school—on and on the talk went, with plenty of prideful interspersions by me about my own affairs at school, affairs that were mostly scholastic, not social. All the while I would be cudgeling my mind for any bit of information I had forgotten to ask about, any precious nugget left buried.

These times at home were intervals of delirious happiness for me, delirious in the literal sense of unreality. There was always the underlying sadness in the knowledge that it could not last, that I must leave again, that I should always be leaving again, that I should never be coming back to stay. On several occasions this sadness was almost unendurable, and I was at the point of refusing to leave, knowing at the same time that if I had not been permitted to go I should have been numb with shock and disappointment. Surely never before were hope and despair so closely akin!

Thus high school was for me the closing of the door on the Dakota I had known, the beginning of a permanent leave-taking. After the first few of these weekend returns I was aware that something had changed for me, something was lost, irretrievably, and this awareness was a large part of the underlying sadness. Identifying, analyzing, understanding this loss was a slow and painful process for it was no trival matter. It encompassed all the ethereal fantasies that had buoyed up my spirit during the homesteading venture. What dreams my brothers and I had shared! We would enact our own Swiss Family Robinson saga here on the prairie. We would build our own empire with its rich farms and herds, and become famous throughout the land as entrepreneurs of the New West. Mother and father would come to visit us, aglow with pride over our fat cattle, sleek horses, substantial buildings, bountiful crops—our entire thrifty, well-managed, successful entourage. In short, they would be proud of us! On and on the dreams went, enough to fill several lifetimes.

Now, in me, I knew these dreams were dead. New ones were sprouting in their place, it is true, but in these I was not united with the rest of my family as before. These new dreams had taken a different direction, so different that the others could no longer be at the heart of them, only on the periphery. At times I was sad and remorseful, and tried to root them out, to return myself to the tight encompassing of my family, but it was no use. Ah, Thomas Wolfe! I did not know you then, but when you told me later, "You can't go home again," I knew immediately what you meant.

After this there came a period of some years (1917–1923) when I scarcely thought of South Dakota at all. I became engulfed in medical school, eyes glued to books and microscopes; long hours in laboratories, hospital wards, and out-patient cubicles. There was little time for daydreaming, star-gazing, or backward musings. Not until I was married and our three children were born, as I have said in the Preface, did the Dakota memories begin burgeoning, always stimulated by contacts with my brothers and sisters and their families.

Just two years short of the fiftieth anniversary of our first arrival, the five of us made a pilgrimmage back to the old homestead. "We should come back again in '59," Floyd said, with his customary exuberance. "That will be fifty years." But I think we all knew we should not be coming back; that this was the final farewell.

We chose a good year for it, as it happened. There had been plenty of rain. The crops were flourishing, the pastures green, the cattle looked well fed. We all felt lighthearted as we drove along. The most startling change in the landscape was that there were full-grown trees in some places. At one spot where we crossed a creek over a little wooden bridge, willows and cottonwoods grew tall enough to shade the road.

We stopped at the old schoolhouse, and went inside. I had taught here the year after I finished high school and I looked about, foolishly hopeful of finding some memento of my tenure—the "Song of the Lark" hanging on the wall, or *Gulliver's Travels, Oliver Twist,* or *Poems Every Child Should Know,* on the bookshelves, all things I had bought with money from a box supper. None of these remained, however. With a little thrill of excitement I picked up a brass hand-bell sitting on the dusty desk. Probably this was the very one I had used! There was nothing about it to deteriorate, as books and pictures may. I clanged it once, and set it down again. It sounded like a knell.

Now we drove a half-mile south to the homestead, the end point of our pilgrimmage. The house was unchanged except for aging, and the paint was entirely gone. A young girl of about fourteen years came to the door and invited us in. She was the only one at home. Her mother was attending Teachers' Institute in Winner, she said, preparatory to teaching in the fall in the schoolhouse we had just left. We sat for awhile in the tiny living room, but found little to talk about. The thoughts of each of us seemed to smother words. I glanced repeatedly at our girl-hostess. "That could be I," I kept thinking. As we left I thrust a bill into her hand. A token blessing? Or a petal of remembrance for my own past? It was probably a little of both.

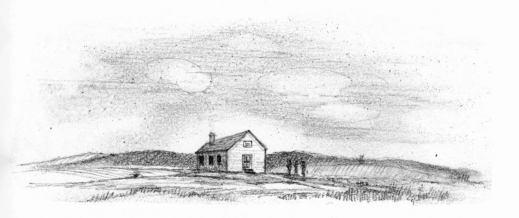